HOW I BECAME THE FITTEST WOMAN ON EARTH

Always believe in yourself.

Keep on trying because something great will come from constantly grinding and striving to be the best version of yourself.

First published in Australia by BL Southwick Publishing Pty Ltd

ACN 624 447 874

Front cover art photographed by Wes Nel
Design and layout by Krys Angeles (Darwin Life Pty Ltd)
All internal photographs courtesy Tia-Clair Toomey unless otherwise credited
Tia-Clair Toomey, Author
Kaia Wright, Co-Author
Beth Ruge, Editor

ISBN 978-0-646-98727-9

MY STORY SO FAR

TIA-CLAIR TOOMEY

How I Became The Fittest Woman On Earth

BL Southwick Publishing Pty Ltd

CONtents

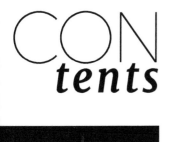

INTRODUCTION

"How did you win the CrossFit Games?"

As you can imagine, I get asked this question a lot. In fact, I get asked this question at least twice a day. Now, before you turn the pages of this book and get stuck into my story, I'll tell you right now - I don't have the answer. I wish I could give you the golden ticket or a magic formula that assures you one of the 40 coveted spots at the CrossFit Games but I can't. What I can give you, is an open and honest account of my life so far and the things I've learnt along the way.

I know I'm still young and some people might question why I'm writing a book so early in my career. The reason is, I believe I have a story worth sharing and what better time to share my story than now - while I'm at the top of my game.

I got to achieve my two dreams of going to the Olympics for weightlifting and standing on the number one podium at the 2017 CrossFit Games and what I know is this; it took a hell of a lot of self-belief, determination and hard work, a commitment to enjoying the journey and a mantra of being better than yesterday. In this book, I will share my story, along with all the little things that help me get better every day - the food I eat, the way I think and the training programs I follow, all of which have helped me to become the best.

When I look back on everything I've done, I can see why I am where I am and all the poignant moments and people in my life that have helped me to get here. My upbringing on the farm, my parents who taught me to work hard, my coaches and mentors who guided and believed in me, the naysayers who gave me the drive to prove people wrong and my secret weapon, coach and husband Shane, who inspires me to achieve every day. These things and these people are the ingredients in my recipe for success.

If you're not willing to hook in and push that little bit harder and faster, you won't get there and out of everything, I think it's my never-say-die attitude that gets me over the line every time. Nobody else can take you to the place you want to end up. You have to get there yourself.

This book begins with my primary school years as a 10-year-old living on a cane farm in Queensland and finishes with my win at the 2017 CrossFit Games. It isn't a traditional life story that includes all the fine details, but rather a selection of memories that have shaped my life and led me to become the Fittest Woman on Earth.

CHAPTER 1

Farm Kid

I was born in Nambour on the 22nd of July 1993 and grew up on a sugarcane farm on Queensland's Sunshine Coast. I am the daughter of Debbi and Brendon Toomey and big sister to Elle and Molly Toomey.

I attended North Arm Primary, an awesome little community school. Unfortunately, though, like most schools, it had its bullies, and the bullies liked picking on me. I don't know why exactly I was a target. When I ask Mum now, she puts it down to jealousy because I was very sporty and did well at running. I guess you could also put it down to the fact that I was pretty different and didn't grow up like most kids.

My family home was located in Dunethin Rock on the Maroochy River. This particular area of coastal Queensland is strongly influenced by sugarcane farming and most people in the region live and breathe an agricultural way of life. Our farm backed onto a beautiful lush riverbank and our house, which was more like a fancy corrugated iron shed, was also Dad's work and storage shed for all the farming equipment. Our family's living quarters were on the top level with a beautiful deck overlooking the river and farm land. My Nan and Pop, my Dad's parents, lived across the main road which was one and a half kilometres away from us. My driveway was very long.

My Mum, Debbi, is a creative woman who loves her cooking, lead lighting and gardening. Thanks to Mum, the property was perfectly groomed with beautiful green grass, big orange and lemon trees, garden beds cornered by rustic sleepers and a little jetty with steps down to the water. Pelicans, ducks and black swans were always around, cruising the waterways. It was a natural oasis.

I had to be creative when I was younger because my sisters didn't come along until I was seven years old, so I was an only child for quite some time. Looking back now, I was definitely a bit on the wacky side. I pretended my dogs were royalty and dressed them up with flowers, collected empty beer cans and cashed them in at the tip and drove around on my red Fergie tractor, helping Dad at work.

As farmers, my parents lead very physically demanding lives. They worked nonstop on the land; clearing, planting and cutting cane ready for the local sugarcane mill in the nearby town of Nambour. The healthy lifestyle of living and working outside gave me and my two younger sisters, Elle and Molly, an awesome start to life.

Mum and Dad never did anything by the book, so we were a pretty unconventional family to say the least. It was the morning of my tenth birthday and I walked into the kitchen to the smell of browning butter. Mum was cooking something special and Dad had just walked in the door from an early morning of work on the tractor.

"T, your Mum and I have been talking and we think it would be great for you to make your own way to and from school in the morning now that you're old enough. We've looked at the bus route and if you get the tinny from our jetty and drive it down the river across to the other side of the bank and moor up at Ozzie's jetty, then you can make the school bus pick up on the other side."

"REALLY? That's the best idea ever!"

I burst with excitement and couldn't wait to tell the kids at school all about it. I scoffed down my food, stuffed my gear in my bag and was out the door in seconds. And that's what I did every day to get to school. I ran from the house down to the jetty, jumped in the tinny and drove across to the other side of the river, skipped up the big hill of our neighbour's farm and got the bus to school. If I wasn't mucking around on the boat or following Dad around on the tractor, I was swimming up and down the Maroochy River with Mum and exploring the property on my quad bike – it didn't get much better for a farm kid.

***

Towards the end of grade five, my school sports teacher, Gwyn, encouraged my friends and I to get into school cross-country. I was naturally athletic and extremely competitive, so I was excited to give cross-country a go. I admired Gwyn and was so thankful for the joy he brought into my life. He made playing sport fun and set me challenges and goals to achieve.

Gwyn looked like a stereotypical hippy, an extremely fit and lean hippy at that. His limbs were long and completely ripped, he wore rainbow tie-dyed t-shirts, had a peace sign tattooed onto his heel and rocked long blonde hair. He always got me and my friends involved in local running events all over the Sunshine Coast. One of my favourites was called the King of the Mountain. The 4.2 kilometre running race is one of the biggest events on the Sunshine Coast's sporting calendar and attracts people from all over the world. Competitors are challenged to run up the face of Mount Cooroora, an extremely steep mountain track that is practically vertical in places.

I dreamed that one day I would be as fit as Gwyn, so I could win Pomona and be crowned Queen of the Mountain! Gywn put together teams of kids from school and helped us train for a 1500 metre fun relay race. We all cheered him on in the morning and then he helped us warm up for our event in the afternoon. The whole day was so much fun, I loved competing and the team atmosphere even more.

I attended every single sports lesson, athletics and cross-country training session just wanting to get better and better. Mum and Dad signed me up to the Sunshine Coast Cross Country Club and Gwyn ran with me every fortnight on a Sunday, so I could build my racing experience. I trained my little arse off but when it came time to perform, I always came second. I would get so frustrated because I knew I could do better.

The silver lining came in grade six at my very first cross-country carnival when I made it to the next stage of competition at Regionals. It was my first time running in a serious event. I was excited and knew I deserved to be there after all my training but didn't know who the competition was or how I'd stack up. The hard work paid off and I placed second, qualifying for the Sunshine Coast team to compete a month later in Brisbane at the State Championships. I didn't do too well and ended up placing eleventh but after that event, that was it. I knew I had found what I wanted to do; compete.

In Australia, the school cross-country and athletics qualification process goes like this; the girls and boys who come first and second at their school carnival progress to Districts, first and second at Districts then progress to Regionals, then the top five at Regionals progress to the State Championships. Then top five again at State Championships progress to National All Schools.

The time came around for the Districts Athletics Carnival and Mum and I headed to Sippy Downs on the Sunshine Coast. I was fidgeting in my seat, itching with excitement! I couldn't wait to race in the 400, 800 and 1500 metres and compete again.

Mum tried to amp me up some more by quoting lines from our favourite movies. The movie 'Gallipoli' was always a crowd pleaser in our household and I knew the words inside and out because Mum and Dad had said them in front of me over a hundred times.

"Alright T, tell me how fast can you run?"
"As fast as a leopard."
"Come on now, tell me, how fast are you going to run?!"
"As fast as a leopard!"
"Then let's see you do it!"

I felt ready to race and could feel the nerves in my belly building into adrenaline.

I was in awe of the atmosphere at Sippy Downs Stadium. It was the first time I'd been to a real athletics facility with a synthetic surface and proper lighting. The nervous energy was pumping through the air and I was lapping up every single second of it.

It's like I feed off competitive environments and my body just kicks into a whole other gear I never knew existed. My race came around and I was able to forget about everything in the past and take things to that next level. I absolutely blitzed my 800 and 1500 metres, finally beating girls I never thought I was capable of overtaking. I placed second overall, which meant I qualified for Regionals.

By the time Regionals came around, I was ready to rumble again, and my time got me through to the State Championships in Brisbane at the QEII Stadium. I think Mum and Dad were as surprised as I was that I had done so well in both cross-country and athletics, mainly because I hadn't done much extra training outside of school.

"You're doing really well, Tia, you gave all those city slickers a run for their money." Mum and I were debriefing on the day and I couldn't stop smiling.

"You've gotten through just on natural talent, T, so imagine what you could do with some training and technique."

'Yeah, just imagine,' I thought. I always wanted to go to the Olympics and in that moment, I believed that maybe I could one day.

"If you really want to do this, then you need to get up and start training before school. But your Dad and I won't be there getting you out of bed each morning, you have to drive it."

She sounded stern but supportive. I knew that my parents would only help me if they could see I was giving it one hundred and ten percent. It felt good to be backed and I wanted to show them and everyone else that I could really do it and get better. I set my first goal for cross-country of placing in the top five at States in July the following year. States were held in a little town called Maryborough, located on the Mary River in Queensland, about three hours north of where we lived.

"Yep, I'm keen, Mum. I want this."

Time waits for no one, so the very next morning at 4.30 am my alarm clock went off and Dad and I got changed and grabbed the measuring tape from the shed. I had always been a morning person, but this was taking it to another level of early.

We walked the perimeter of the headland on our property, marking out 400, 800 and 1500 metres with spray paint. I had butterflies in my tummy. It felt like the beginning of something great.

CHAPTER 2

Fire in my Belly

I got up early every morning from then on. I would warm up first before getting into my session which usually consisted of five sets of 800 metres with a three-minute rest in between, followed by four sets of 200 metres with a three-minute rest in between. My goal would be to beat the times of the first set in my second set.

"How'd I go?"

I'd finish my lap and turn straight to Dad and ask these three words after every run on repeat. I wasn't satisfied unless I was improving my time each crack on the track. We would mix it up with different running distances and Dad would record my times as we went.

Some days, when my legs were completely gone, Dad would surprise me with an extra bit of training. About two weeks into our new program, he threw me a challenge. We had gone harder than ever before, and my sweat was mixing in with the rain pouring down around me. I had wobbly legs where your knees feel like they are about to give in.

"Jog down to the water, T, and do six up and backs across the width of the river to flush out all that lactic acid, then you're done."

I was tired, but my body kicked into 'just do, don't think' mode so down I ran. I muddled my way through the laps, splashing around, but got there in the end and hopped out of the water. A huge smile beamed across my face.

"Do you know what!? That was actually fun as! Thanks for getting me to do that."

Suddenly, I wasn't tired anymore, I just felt high on life. Nothing made me feel as good as I did when I exercised, I couldn't get enough of it.

Dad would do the morning trainings with me and Mum would drive me an hour and a half to the proper track at the University of the Sunshine Coast every Thursday night, where I would receive athletics coaching from an Australian Olympic hurdles coach, Jackie Byrnes. She would help me with the technical aspects of running that Mum and Dad didn't know much about. My parents were really good at reaching out to networks of coaches who lived nearby so I could get access to better training. I look back now at all of the time they put into me and the financial cost of it all and think, 'Wow, I can't believe my parents did that just for me.'

Sport was something I really enjoyed at school, but I always struggled a bit in the classroom. I saw a speech therapist as a young kid and reading and maths certainly weren't my strong points so Mum used cooking as a way for me to improve my learning.

"Alright, here's the recipe - now I want you to grab a bowl and put two and a half cups of coconut milk in here using a one cup, quarter cup and half cup measurement."

"Why does everything always have to be about learning? I just want to sit down and eat already and not have to count and play stupid games every single time. It's dumb!"

I would get frustrated so easily because it was such a simple concept and I just couldn't wrap my head around it. I know Mum was just trying to help but it was the last thing I felt like doing and I could never get the measurements right. The rest of my family paid for my mathematical downfalls. They tasted some interesting interpretations on recipes over the years, thanks to my measuring skills, or lack of!

We all sat down for dinner one night and Mum and Dad ran some new ideas past me.

"Tia, what are your thoughts on joining Nippers and doing surf lifesaving? If you want to take your running to the next level then Dad and I reckon doing something like that will really help with your fitness and conditioning."

When Mum said it was something her and Dad did when they were my age and I'd get to race against kids from out of town I was sold on the idea.

"So, what do you reckon, have a go?" Dad asked.

"Yeah, that would be sick! I wonder how fast I'll be compared to the other girls in the water?"

***

Nippers is a sport for kids aged five to fourteen where they have fun while taking part in 'tests' in the areas of swimming, board paddling and beach sprints.

In 2005, at the end of grade seven, I started my new hobby. I did Nippers alongside cross-country, athletics, netball and tennis. I joined the Mooloolaba Surf Club, perched right on the edge of the Pacific Ocean. I wasn't too great at it, but I did well enough to go to the State Competition held at Kings Beach in Caloundra, an area known for some amazing surf.

It was a clear day, but the waves were huge. Most of the kids pulled out of the event except a handful of the more experienced swimmers. Kids were getting smashed from the waves and thrown all over the place. I was standing next to Dad and another girl I didn't know. Her Dad came up behind us with her change of clothes.

"There is no way you're going out in that, I think we should call it a day."

He made it sound like a tsunami was approaching.

I felt a bit queasy in the guts. I looked over to Dad, expecting him to tell me to pack my bags.

"You ready to rock and roll, T?! Go on, off you go, get out there and show them what you've got!"

Dad sounded so sure, but I certainly wasn't.

"Dad – I don't – I don't know if I can,"
I stuttered and started to step backwards.

"What do you mean, T? Yes, you can! It's not hard, you've just got to swim out there then turn around and come back to shore – simple."
I didn't want to disappoint Dad and thought, 'Don't be so pathetic, Tia, just harden up and at least have a go.' So out I went.

I managed to reach the turnaround mark, but it took me a lot longer than expected. I was getting knocked around pretty bad so I grabbed onto the floating buoy and held my hand up to be rescued by the red rubber ducky. I returned to the shore reasonably unscathed with no fuss or bother from Dad.

"Well, that was an adventure, wasn't it?"

I scrunched my face up.

"I guess you could say that."

We jumped in the car and headed home. It was a pretty silent car ride, because my mind was going a hundred miles an hour.

"Hey Dad, I know I'm already doing running training but can I join the local swimming club as well? I want to become a stronger swimmer. I felt silly out there with that happening to me."

"Great idea, T. Let's see what we can sort out."

Dad was so awesome like that, he was all for me trying everything and nothing was ever too hard. Three days later, I swapped out my early morning runs with 5 am swims and moved my training with Dad to the afternoons.

The fitter I got and the more I succeeded with my sports, the more I realised I didn't need anyone else's approval. I just wanted to be the best I could be. My goal was to make the State Titles and get to the All Schools Nationals and I felt like it was possible. I had finally found my groove and headed into grade eight feeling invincible!

***

Mum reckons that people would pull her aside when I was growing up and say that I was going places. I don't know how people could say that about a short, frizzy-haired girl from the country but looking back, I guess they were onto something. That sort of flattery used to go in one ear and out the other with Mum and Dad. As long as I was happy and healthy, that's all they really cared about.

July 2006 came around, as did the State Titles in Maryborough, and I came through with a third place! I had never felt anything like it; I couldn't believe I had come eleventh the year before and only a year later, got to stand on the podium. I was actually getting somewhere and achieving!

I couldn't wipe the grin off my face, it felt like the best day ever.

One thing I did start to notice was that I had a different attitude to the girls I was competing against. I trained and competed to get better and winning was secondary for me. A lot of the other girls just wanted to win, win, win and if they lost too many times they'd just give up. Sure, winning felt great but that wasn't where I got the most kicks, I loved seeing myself improve. Even when I won races at school or at the local competitions, I was still determined to get a faster time the next time around.

If I lost a race and started to sulk, I'd get shut down pretty quick smart by Dad.

"Don't get upset. Reflect and think about what you did to prepare for that race and what you could do better next time. What did you eat, how much sleep did you get and how hard did you train? I bet there is always an area you can improve on."

This was drummed into me from a young age and it just clicked for me. I think you've got to have some bad runs to appreciate the good ones. When you're young, you can't always have a winning streak. It doesn't prepare you enough. You learn more from your losses then you do your wins. For the majority of my childhood and teenage years, I never had a winning streak. I was always chasing someone, always the bridesmaid, so to speak.

My athletics coach, Jackie, gave me her book; Running Fast: Coaching Tips for Young Athletes, Coaches, Teachers and Parents. I read the book every day in the lead-up to Nationals, taking notes and telling my parents all the things I was learning. I felt so fit and so strong and I couldn't wait to compete. Mum and I flew down to Adelaide in South Australia. It was the first time I had been on a trip outside of Queensland and I was so excited to be going on a plane. I thought I was such a big girl and was so happy to spend some special time with Mum. We went and had a look around the beautiful city while Dad phoned in from work, making sure I was stopping to stretch and eat the right food. The night before my race, Mum massaged my legs and Dad talked me through what I needed to do the next day to get in the zone.

The morning of the Nationals, I had that breathless nervous feeling building in my belly. While most of the athletes were warming up, I was in the bathroom being sick. I've learned a couple of tricks to manage my nerves over the years, but it's usually a good sign when I feel that way. I always seem to compete better when I'm nervous, especially when I get teary. As soon as I feel tears welling, I know I'm going to perform.

This particular morning, I didn't have tears. I was nervous, shaking, almost convulsing, a complete mess. I couldn't enjoy the experience because my emotions were all over the shop. It threw me a little bit but I ended up running a personal best, placing sixth overall and was the first Queenslander over the line. It was a pivotal moment for me because it taught me about coping with pressure and being able to perform when the stakes a high.

After the fun of Nationals, I was on top of the world but a part of me wondered whether my performance was beginner's luck. Nonetheless, I was happy with my new passion and felt like my life really had some meaning.

It was nearing the end of the school year and the end of primary school for me. It was a sticky hot weekend and Gwyn took me and some kids from school to the nearby Eumundi Markets to celebrate.

"Tia, your running has gotten really good. You have natural talent and are improving all the time. Do you enjoy doing it?"

"Yeah, of course Gwyn!"

I bounced right back at him.

"Well, you've ticked the first box. You've found something you are good at and you love doing. You may not see it for yourself yet, but there's something very special about you, Tia, you're set for big things."

I thought, 'Well, if someone as fit as Gwyn thinks I'm okay at running, then I must be half decent. I mean, not everyone can make Nationals in a sport that they've only done seriously for a year.'

CHAPTER 3
Family is Everything

I hear stories of athletes who come from broken families and poor living conditions who still go on to achieve amazing things. I admire them a lot because I doubt I would be where I am if it wasn't for the undivided attention and investment from my loved ones. I'm very lucky; the support from my family is the fuel that keeps me going.

I know people say clichéd things all the time about how thankful they are for their family's support, so those sorts of statements can lose their meaning. But honestly, I can't say enough how lucky I am to have the strong family network that I do.

My parents didn't have any time for themselves when I was a kid because they worked so hard on the cane farm for Nan and Pop. Somehow, they still managed to create incredible opportunities for me to experience and learn new things.

My Mum is a strong and independent woman who is hands-down the hardest worker I know. Everything she does is geared towards creating the best opportunities for me and my sisters and she is our biggest protector. Mum's 'never say die' attitude has rubbed off on me and my sisters. If I'd lose a race she'd say, 'That's just more ammo for you to work harder next time,' any time I would feel defeated about something, she'd say, 'What's wrong? Do you need a big Mumma bear hug?" And if I ever used the word 'can't', she'd give me the good old, 'There's no such thing as can't.'

My Dad is calm and centred and has a way of making me feel safe. His voice on the end of the phone saying, 'You'll be right,' is all I need when I'm feeling unsure. As a kid, Dad always held me accountable when it came to my training but managed to do it in a way where I never felt pressured. It was Dad's commitment to get up with me every morning that gave me the motivation to train harder – for me and for him.

I loved my childhood, but it did get lonely at times. I asked my parents non-stop for years if I could have a brother or a sister and when I was six years old, my wish finally came true. It seemed like Elle was in Mum's belly for eternity but when the day came for me to go into the hospital and meet her, I made a big fuss with Nan because everything had to be perfect.

"Nan, can we go past my house, so I can pick up my present? I need to give Elle a gift."

Nan just gave me one of her 'okay love' looks and pulled into our driveway. I jumped out of the car and bolted straight into to my room. I pulled out my collection of 33 teddy bears and deliberated over which one to give to her. It took me so long to decide, because I loved every single teddy and I didn't want to give Elle one that I might want to play with again but didn't want to give her a bad one either. I finally made up my mind and skipped back to the car.

"Nan, I LOVE Elle so much that I have chosen to give her my favourite Bunny teddy!" It was such a big deal to me. I took the role of being an older sister very seriously. This care and love carried on as Elle grew up and then when my second sister Molly came along three years later, that was just the cherry on top.

Given the age difference between my sisters and I, I have always felt like they are my own children in a way. I want them to look up to me, so I constantly try to better myself and show them that anything is possible if they set their minds to it. I don't know if it's because all my friends had older brothers or younger sisters that I wanted siblings or whether I just liked the idea of having mini-mes. But whatever it was, I finally felt whole when they came along. I entertained myself for hours playing games with them, pretending I was their mum or treating them like real-life dolls. I would dress them up, strap them into the back of my toy tractor and take them on adventures all over our property. Mum says it's a wonder we're all still alive because of the misadventures we had together.

I'll never forget when Elle almost drowned. It was a rainy grey day and Mum, Elle and I were driving the dingy across the river. I was steering the boat and just happened to turn around. Behind me, I saw a ring ripple in the water and looked back to the boat and screamed.

"Mum, where's Elle!?"

There were little gumboots left in the same position where three-year-old Elle was sitting moments earlier. Mum saw the ring and dived into the cold water to rescue her. Elle was still conscious, and we got her straight up onto the boat and into the warm house. Living on the farm and thinking we were invincible lead to some very close mishaps.

***

My grandparents on both sides of my family were a huge part of my life growing up and I spent a lot of my time hanging out with them on the weekends. Disey and Pa would watch most of my running events and Nan and Pop would take me to most of my training sessions.

My Pop was a very special man, everything about him was just so loveable. He was my hero. He had a soft and sensitive soul but a hard exterior. I felt like I could get away with anything with him. He loved giving me a big hug every time he saw me, but he could never wrap his arms all the way around because his hard pot belly would get in the way.

I admired Pop's work ethic. His body was covered with scars and blemishes from a life of working outdoors. All over his skin he had bumps, bruises and burns. They were his badges of honour from years of cutting cane in the elements. It was Pop who taught me about physical and mental strength. He would always say to me, You may be strong, but are you tough?'

School holidays had just begun, and I went around to Pop's for tea and biscuits.

"Pop, you know how you always talk about being tough, is it better to be strong or tough?"

"Put it this way, I may not have been as strong as some of the other workers on the cane farm, but I worked harder, faster and smarter because I knew my family depended on me."

I thought Pop was like a wise old wizard. He said everything with such thought and consideration.

"The strength of the mind beats the strength of the body every time. You can always outwork the strongest man in the room if his mind is weaker than yours."

I hung onto Pop's every word and those words stuck with me more than any others. I ran straight back home.

"Mum, Mum, do you think I'm tough?"

"I don't say that you've got the Heart of Valour for nothing."

My whole body filled with pride. The fact my Mum and Pop thought I was tough meant everything to me.

Looking back, I can really see what Pop means now. People confuse toughness with strength all the time. You can lift all the weights in the world but that doesn't mean you're capable of digging deep physically and mentally at crunch time.

To me, toughness is the ability to perform, regardless of the circumstances. If someone is willing to have the patience and stay positive and focused no matter how many times shit hits the fan, they will have the edge over the others.

It was Pop who took me to swimming lessons every morning. He would pick me up at 4 am and get me to the pool, ready for my training. We would have so many fun times in the car on the way.

"Pop, why do you always drive so close to the line on the road when we turn a corner?"

"Well, do you ever see racehorses taking their turns wide on the track? No, I don't think you do. They take every turn tight to make sure they get every advantage possible. I do it with my driving to save time and fuel and you can do it with your running too."

I just giggled at his farfetched explanation. I knew it was because Pop was getting old and couldn't see very well, but nonetheless it was a good story and I went along with him.

Pop would sit at the pool with his newspaper waiting for me to finish my four-kilometre swim with the rest of the squad. Then I'd get dressed at the pool and Pop would take me to school. We'd do that same routine every morning except for Saturday and Sunday.

I ask myself sometimes why I'm so driven. Or people ask me 'what is your why?' I think it comes down to wanting to make my family proud. My Disey would always say that no matter what it was, when

I had something I wanted to achieve, no one was going to get in my way. My determination has been fierce from a very young age and I have always set goals with my family alongside me. And as soon as I have something in mind, that's it. I am unstoppable.

CHAPTER 4
Big Changes

The sugarcane mill in Nambour shut down in 2004, so people started clearing out to find work elsewhere. Dad is a plumber by trade, so he did some plumbing work up north until he secured a more permanent job as a diesel fitter on one of the mines. One day, he arrived home after working away and sat everyone down in the living room.

"Looks like we've got a new adventure ahead of us. We'll be moving in a couple of months."

I was confused and didn't quite comprehend what he was saying.

"I've found a good job in Weipa where I've been working for the past four months. It's a small mining town of about 3,000 people, at the top of the Cape York Peninsula in Queensland. T, you can finish off the first term of grade eight here and then we'll head up."

Still no words, just complete shock, I couldn't believe it.

I moped around the farm for the next few weeks feeling sorry for myself but it was two days before the big move when I finally lost it. I felt short-changed. I couldn't believe I had to say goodbye to Nippers and swimming, the two things I had begun to love and get good at, and to all my friends.

"Mum, my life is over. I am never going to be happy again, it's not fair."

I was pretty good at dramatising situations and this was no exception.

"Change is as good as a holiday, T, there will be new opportunities for you where we're heading."

'Opportunities in an isolated mining town known for its extreme humidity and cyclones, as if, Mum.' I wanted to say what I was thinking but I bit my tongue.

"Yeah, I guess."

I didn't sound at all convinced.

Nan and Pop sold their house and moved into our house. The rest of us packed up shop and drove 1,500 miles north, ready for a new life.

After five long days, we arrived at our new home. It was located in the middle of the small town, across the road from the only school and an Australian Rules football oval. We had neighbours for the first time ever which I thought was cool and after a few weeks I started to open my eyes to the new possibilities.

I did the last half of grade eight at Western Cape College where I got right back into my sport and all the school's outdoor activities. Disey and Pa called up after my first week of school.

"How'd it go, love?"

"You wouldn't believe it, but I'm loving school! I've found a running group and started playing touch footy."

"That's good to hear my love, and remember to do your homework!"

"Of course, Disey!"

I didn't really listen to the bit about homework - anything to do with school work went in one ear and out the other. It's not that I was naughty, I still tried my best in the classroom, I just preferred to be outside playing sport. I did cross-country and athletics in the afternoons and swam in the mornings at a pool close to home. For a small town, Weipa had lots of sporting activities for people to get involved in. There was a fishing competition, a mixed touch football series, an annual bull riding event and a triathlon race. If I wasn't playing sport I was out bush, having fun. Dad worked shift work so on his days off, my family and I got to go fishing, camping and motorbike riding. My sisters and I were really spoilt.

***

Dad came home from his shift and told me to get changed and we headed across to the football oval.

"Alright, T, let's mark out our track so we can keep up your training, you've got some comps coming up."

We walked around the oval and marked out 400 metres, just like old times. I got back into my training groove, following the same programs I did on the farm. I made the State Championships, but for the Peninsula Team this time. Dad and I travelled down to Townsville and competed in the four-kilometre cross-country race. I did worse than I expected, placing fifth, I was disappointed and dissatisfied.

"Hey Dad, do you think we could try and find me a coach for my running like what I used to do with Jackie? I want some more help with technique and strategies."

Dad was all over it and before I knew it, I started training with a running coach from Brisbane named John Clancy, who still programs for my sister Molly today. John is a kind man who was always encouraging me and forever trying to make me laugh. He had terrible Dad jokes but I really liked him, and he knew what he was doing.

From grade eight to 10 I continued running training at school. I represented the Peninsula region at State Championships and then went on to Nationals, representing Queensland.

Dad trained me based on programs from John Clancy which were always something new and interesting. I missed the regular racing and competitions I got to do when I lived on the Sunshine Coast but through my running and swimming, I kept at it.

Weipa has a monsoonal climate with distinct wet and dry seasons but one thing is for sure, it is always distinctly hot. I was used to the cooler climate in Nambour so it was hard running in Weipa but it definitely conditioned me for exercising in harsh conditions.

My parents put a lot of effort into my training but I noticed myself starting to slowly lose interest. I knew I'd regret it if I quit and I didn't want to let my parents down after everything they'd done for me. I kept on training and decided to enter myself into the local triathlon, Aluminum Man and Woman, during my grade 10 school holidays, just to change things up and keep my training interesting.

I entered the Women's Open category for more competition because there wasn't any competition for me in the younger division and I was the youngest by a country mile. The race started and off we went straight into the water. I was getting nudged and kicked around by the other women, but I pushed through and managed to find my own. I found the swimming easy considering I had only just gotten back into it and I surprised myself by coming out of the water first.

I ran up the passage towards the bikes where competitors were waiting for their team mates. There was no one there for me because I was flying solo in the individual's division. As I ran up to my bike I noticed a guy staring at me, we caught each other's eyes and I looked away with embarrassment.

I hopped on my bike and bolted off. The lactic acid had built up badly in my legs, but the cycle flushed it out and I was ready for the final run. The running leg doubled back on itself and on the way back through, I saw the same guy from the bike area running towards me.

"You can do it, hang on in there, you're almost finished!"

I don't know what gave me the urge to yell out to a stranger, but I liked the look of him. I thought he was pretty cute actually and discovered later that stranger was actually Shane. I won the Women's Open Individual Race and was awarded the Aluminum Woman of the year. Everyone kept on congratulating me like it was some awesome feat but it wasn't any Nationals so I didn't think too much of it.

Shane and I both remember briefly crossing paths that day and look back on it now and laugh. Shane tells me that he tried to impress me by riding his bike as fast as he could to catch up but completely overdid it and couldn't even get close. So, when I called out to him and encouraged him to keep going, he was utterly embarrassed because he was trying so hard to inspire me.

***

Dad and I joined the local gym, so I could start lifting light weights to improve on my power and speed for running. Every now and then I would notice Shane at the gym, but we didn't know each other's names back then. Dad and I went for a Friday night session after dinner and did our last workout for the week ahead of the Weipa Fishing Classic the next day.

The fishing comp is held every year over the June long weekend for three days. People come to Weipa from all over Cape York and interstate to compete for a prize pool of about $100,000. The event has heaps of activities with entertainment and stalls; it's like a mini carnival. I was hanging out with my girlfriends from school when Samantha told me about her boyfriend's mate.

"Tia, Daniel has a friend who wants to meet you. He's seen you around town. He's hot and a little bit older too."

I was quite flattered at the time to think an older guy was interested in getting to know me. Samantha and I walked over to a group of guys I'd never met before.

"Tia, this is Shane, Daniel's friend I was telling you about."

I couldn't believe it, it was the same guy from the gym. I was quietly surprised to see him again.

"Hey, I'm Tia. I've seen you around a few times, nice to meet you."

We got talking and got to know each other a little bit. I told him about my running and how I was training for States and Nationals.

"That's awesome. Well, if your Dad can't train with you some afternoons, let me know and I can help. I don't know too much about running but I'm sure I could start and stop a stopwatch for you."

We exchanged numbers and Shane started timekeeping for me during my training sessions in the afternoon. It was the only way my parents would ever let us hang out, they were quite strict on me dating boys and going to parties. In the afternoons, Shane would knock on my front door to get me for training. Elle, Molly and I would go with Shane across the road to the oval and start my session. I reckon my parents encouraged my sisters to come to training with us because they didn't want Shane and I to be alone.

It's crazy to think that Shane has been a part of my team since I was fourteen. I loved training with him; he was great at encouraging and pushing me to get better. I felt like he really believed in me.

When Shane and I met, we were drawn to each other because we both had ambition and wanted to achieve our goals. I would go to my athletics events and Shane would be so supportive in helping me train to get from Districts, to Regionals, States to Nationals. I was very lucky to find someone so special at such a young age that loved and supported me.

Elle and Molly were at the shops with Mum, so Shane and I trained at the oval by ourselves for my last session before Districts. The sun disappeared, signalling the end of our afternoon training session.

"It's so inspiring to see someone as driven as you, Tia. It's hard for you to grasp because you've always done it, but I don't know any other person who wakes up every single morning at 5 am, swims three kilometres in the pool, goes to school, then comes home and trains for another two hours on the oval. Training is like religion to you, it's pretty amazing."

I was taken aback. I had never heard someone say something so nice to me before. I never really looked at it that way. That ambition and expectation of training double days started from the age of 10 and just came naturally to me, I didn't know any better.

Shane doesn't swim, so I kept swimming with Dad in the mornings at the pool in Weipa. Dad would sit at the end of the pool on a chair and every time I swam to the end, he would give me instructions or words of encouragement. I loved the mornings with Dad. It was our time to connect and hang out together. I really started to fall in love with my new home. Training was good, school was good, I had my family and I had Shane.

***

In 2009, my parents made the decision to enroll me in boarding school at Townsville Grammar for grade eleven and twelve to focus on my education. The school was sixteen hours' drive south of Weipa on the coast of Queensland. The first twelve weeks away from home were the hardest. I cried myself to sleep at night, wishing I was back at home in Weipa with my family and Shane. I was really homesick and it took me a little while to find my feet and get back into sport and the things that made me happy. I had so many opportunities at my fingertips - there was a pool right outside my dorm, a running track on the school oval and lots of team sports available to be a part of. I made amazing friends and had a real sense of independence for the first time in my life. I cried walking into the school the day Dad dropped me off, but I cried even more the day I graduated and drove out of the gates for the last time. I felt empowered and ready to take on the next chapter in my life.

CHAPTER 5

No Direction

I finished school and enrolled in the University of Queensland in Brisbane, so I could be closer to the Sunshine Coast. Shane was based on the Sunshine Coast living with mates, flying in and out of Perth in Western Australia, working as a mechanical fitter on the mines. He worked long hours and made really good money.

I moved into my Auntie's house in Brisbane. I liked the idea of being a midwife but I didn't score well enough in school, so I settled on studying a double Bachelor of Nursing and Exercise and Movement Science. It was nothing like what I expected; I didn't enjoy it and just went through the motions. I wanted to get back into my running, but I couldn't find the motivation. I felt like that ship had sailed and I was too old to go any further. I signed up to a local gym where I did Les Mills classes a few times a week and when Shane came home from his swing, we lifted weights together. Other than that, I filled my days with half-arsed study for university and shit-kicking around my Auntie's place. I felt like a failure.

Shane's contract was for three years and he still had two more to go. I thought it was ridiculous that I was finally out of school and we couldn't even live together, let alone see each other! I stayed at university for another six months but became progressively more and more disinterested. It was 11 pm on a Friday night and after a three-hour anatomy lecture, I made the long journey home on the bus. I called Shane and told him I just wasn't interested in studying anymore. The whole 'go to university, work hard, save money, buy a house and live happily ever after' thing wasn't working for me. The formula I grew up believing in didn't seem to be delivering the fulfillment I had hoped.

"What's gotten into you, Tia? It's not like you to give up. There's nothing over here for you in Perth and I'm thinking of quitting anyway. Why don't I pack up here and with the money I've saved, I'll buy us a place in Brisbane so we're still close to our family and friends?"

Shane's decisiveness helped put things back on track and kept my emotions at bay for the time being. He bought a house and saw out his last couple of months at his job. Our first home was a beautiful Queenslander, with a blue and white weatherboard exterior and tin roof. It was only tiny, but it had two sweet balconies off the porch, three little rooms and a funky black tile bathroom. We created a warm home and loved having our own space. I was on uni break, trying to decide whether to defer my studies; I literally felt like my life was going backwards.

I had too much time on my hands to think. I would lie in bed and examine my life, overthinking all the various life paths in front of me. Each path looked worse than the other, stopping me from moving forward with anything. My anxiety was heightened by the increasing uncertainty in my life, especially the unpredictability of where Shane and I would get our next jobs and what sort of career I wanted to pursue. I complained to Shane that I was bored and lonely, and I could tell he was getting over it. I was over myself, so I can't imagine how he felt. One day, I came home from the shops after lunch. Shane was standing in the hallway beaming and out ran the cutest little dog I have ever seen.

"I had to do something to stop you complaining about being bored. Now you have a job on your hands looking after this little one. She's a red Staffy."

I turned into a complete ball of moosh over her, she was adorable. We named her Rhi Rhi, she was my little baby and kept me occupied while Shane was away finishing things up in Perth.

It's pretty embarrassing but I can't believe how lazy and spoilt I became. I just sat at home and hung out with my dog while Shane supported us both. And when I wanted my first car, Nan, Dad's Mum, bought me one. Everything came easy. I was so totally spoilt it makes me sick thinking about it now.

"Make sure you don't tell your parents I bought you this, I will be hung out to dry. I've always wanted to get you your first car, so I'm going to follow through with it but make sure you start looking for a job soon."

It's not that I was inherently lazy and liked doing nothing, I think it came down to the fact that I just didn't know what I wanted to do with my life. Committing to a career has always been a really important decision for me because the rest of your life is a very long time.

After working a crappy nightshift job in Brisbane for a month, Shane secured a great paying job working for a mining company in Gladstone, a small city home to a large multi-commodity shipping port. We packed up all our stuff in an old white Mercedes van and drove up in September 2011. It was a draining six-hour drive, but we made it in the end and Shane started working immediately on a Monday to Friday roster. Everyone described Gladstone as a gritty industrial town with no heart and nothing to do and my first impression wasn't far off from that.

We were put into a very basic transitional home until we found a place to rent. It was a typical brick suburban home, in one of those old housing developments where the houses are so close, you may as well be living with your neighbours.

I didn't defer university until Shane got the confirmation of the job in Gladstone. I always made sure I didn't give up on something unless I had something else to replace it with and I secured a job in Gladstone as a dental assistant. For our first Christmas in Gladstone, Shane bought me another dog as a surprise so Rhi Rhi had a companion. I woke up on Christmas morning to a beautiful white Labrador puppy with a tiny red collar, who we named Sam. He was so adorable and became my running buddy. For 18 months, I worked from Monday to Friday and Shane continued working for Rio Tinto as a mechanical fitter. Life was so simple. We went to work, came home, went out and socialised with new friends over pizza, Mexican or Thai food once a week. Life started turning around for me, but it definitely wasn't what I had expected to be doing when I was growing up. I always thought I would at least be working towards a goal.

We went to the gym every morning at 5 am before our work. Shane was always good at correcting my posture and pushing me to push myself.

"Tense your abs, push for four more reps. I know you've got it in you."

"Arghhhh!"

I pumped through the pain of my last few back squats. I always seemed to train better when Shane was around.

"Good session today, Tia, you killed it. Hey, I've been thinking – my work is looking for someone reliable and willing to work night shift. It's a lab technician role. The pay is good, and I reckon you'd be a perfect fit for it. You should apply; I'll help you pull a resume together."

I brushed him off before he could finish his sentence.

"But I don't even have a degree."

"It's not all about degrees. Just apply and see what happens. Look at me, Tia, I don't have a degree. I have a trade and I've had good well-paying jobs since I left school."

If Shane was backing me then I didn't have anything to lose, plus he's not one to pull the wool over my eyes.

I applied for the job at Rio Tinto and I got it. All of a sudden, I felt so proud and so motivated. I called all my family back home to tell them the news. So there I was, signing a contract to an $80,000 a year job with no experience, working half the year because my roster was a five day on, five day off day shift and a four day on, four day off night shift roster on rotation. I'd hit the jackpot.

I was a new person and I had a spring in my step. The hours were tiring but having routine was awesome and the money coming in was a bonus. It was nice to finally pull my weight in our relationship and we started looking for a house in Gladstone to buy together. Life had derailed momentarily but I was back on track and heading upwards.

We planned to work our arses off in Gladstone for five years, save enough money and set ourselves up well before starting a family.

Shane played for the local Rugby Club and was really good at it; his adrenaline after winning a game was contagious. I knew that something was missing in my life and it became obvious. It was my sport.

"After watching you have fun on the field like that, Shane, it makes me miss competing."

"Why don't you get back into your running training and compete in the Women's Opens competitions for athletics? It will be perfect for you, you can train on your days off and I bet you'll surprise yourself with how quickly you can bounce back."

I wanted to get fit, so Shane and I enrolled in mixed netball and touch football teams and started doing running sessions at the local track. I had learnt so much about running and training, so I got out some old programs to follow. I didn't want to train for the 1500 metres or 800 metres anymore so I decided to focus only on the 400 metre hurdles. I joined the Gladstone local athletics club and trained to compete in the regular racing meets on Friday nights.

CHAPTER 6

Game Changer

It's crazy to think that it was only five years ago when I came across the thing that would change my life forever. Shane came home from work one Friday afternoon and told me to get my training gear on, ready for CrossFit.

"Huh? Cross what?" I scrunched up my face.

"Our rugby coach has been making the team go to this CrossFit gym to improve our fitness and it's really making a difference. I met the owner Benito yesterday and he said it would really improve your running too."

Shane had that tone in his voice where I knew he had made his mind up already, so I had no option other than to succumb.

"If you want to compete at State level again, then you need to get fitter and I think this will help."

"Yeah, righto, why not?"

I got my gear on and we were out the door before I could give it any more thought.

I'm not going to sugarcoat it but at first, I bloody hated CrossFit. I would have walked out if Shane didn't know the guys running the class. We pulled into the carpark at CrossFit Gladstone ready for the 6.30 pm class. The gym didn't look like other gyms I had been to before. It was a little bit rough around the edges and was laid out pretty unconventionally. There were ropes and tractor tyres in one corner and random structures built into the walls and ceilings. It looked like a gymnast got together with a weightlifter and together they created their perfect gym.

AC/DC was blaring so loud my eardrums were vibrating and everyone was speaking in what sounded like another language.

"What's your 1RM snatch?"

"I'm not feeling up to snatching today."

"Clean and jerks are my favourite."

I had no idea what they were going on about and even heard two ladies yelling about other women across the floor.

"I love Dianne but hate Fran!"

I was pretty taken aback. I didn't understand who Fran was and why she was being bagged out at the gym.

I smiled at the coach and made out like I was excited to be there because he looked pumped to have new people attend his class.

"Alright guys, welcome to CrossFit Gladstone, my name is Sean and I'm your coach for today's class. If you have any injuries, questions or concerns, please come and see me."

He seemed nice but kind of arrogant at the same time. I don't know what it was, but I just wasn't vibing off his energy or the energy in the room for that matter.

There were a range of numbers up on the white board and Sean demonstrated each exercise in detail.

I was the type of person who just wanted to get in and do the work and figure it out along the way for myself, not have my hand held. One movement that I had never seen before was a handstand push-up and all I wanted to do was try that because it looked really hard. But the coach wouldn't let me do the movement at all.

"Can I just go straight up into a handstand and give it a shot? I reckon I can do it."

"No, I think it's best not to, Tia, let's just stick with the way I suggested for now."

'Pfffft, who is this hero?' I thought to myself. 'I've come here to learn and get better and he's not even letting me do what I want to do and what I know I can do.'

I looked around and everyone - I mean, everyone - was at least in a handstand against the wall and I sure as hell knew I could do that, which made me even more annoyed. I got through the full session but was hardly impressed. I said a forced thank you to Sean and Shane and I got into our car to head home.

"Shane, that was THE WORST idea you've ever had, you couldn't pay me to go back there! Those people are all arrogant and love themselves, what on earth could they teach me?"

Shane let me rant on and on and didn't say much, which usually means he doesn't agree with what I'm saying.

I voiced my opinion with such conviction and hated my experience so much that I honestly can't believe I ended up back there a couple of months later at the start of 2013, paying for a one-month unlimited pass.

As it turned out, I bumped into one of the coaches from CrossFit Gladstone on two different occasions and both times I saw her it was the same thing.

"Tia, great to see you. When are you and Shane coming back? I'm really looking forward to training you. I think you've got some good natural talent there."

Jardan is such a lovely girl and was so warm and genuine to me that I felt bad about not going back to the gym. And when she asked me about it the second time, I got guilt-tripped into signing up. I figured I needed to get off my power trip and give it another try.

For the first week, I felt self-conscious and was so intimidated by everyone that I needed Shane to come with me as my security blanket. I got to know the trainers better and started to warm to them all, but I had my favourites. Jardan and her partner, Nick, were both very experienced Level One CrossFit coaches and were heavily involved with the gym.

They were my first two coaches and it was them that made me feel the most comfortable and welcome.

"We've seen you in action before, Tia, we know what you're capable of and boy, are you strong."

I had no idea what Nick was talking about.

"Jardan and I have both met you before at your old gym and we've watched you lift from afar, we admired your strength. I don't think you realise but you can lift quite a lot for a girl your size."

That was nice to hear but I didn't really agree, and I didn't pay any attention to my training back then.

***

Once I got into CrossFit, I couldn't believe how many people already knew about it and how big the international CrossFit community was. I'd overhear people talking about it in the supermarket, see it on my Facebook feed and read about it in magazines. I started googling articles and reading up on its background and how it all came about.

Its popularity is remarkable, given the first CrossFit gym opened in Seattle not that long ago, in the year 2000. In saying that though, the CrossFit training principles were established over 30 years ago by Greg Glassman, the founder of CrossFit.

A former gymnast, Greg trained in gymnastics and a range of other sports both competitively and for fun, constantly challenging his mates to see who was the fittest. After a few years, he noticed that he could always find a person who was better than him in one sport but not in all sports across the board. He could beat everyone in a bicycle race but would lose in a running race or could squat twice as much as a mate but would be outdone on a bench press.

This concept laid the foundation of CrossFit as it is known today. In the words of Greg himself, CrossFit is about 'people achieving a goal of greater work capacity across broad time and modal domains.' 'Broad time' means at different levels of intensity and 'broad modal domains' refers to a person's general physical skills including cardiovascular and respiratory endurance, stamina, strength, flexibility, power, speed, coordination, agility, balance and accuracy.

In other words, it's cool to be able to throw a barbell around, it's exciting to learn how to do handstand push-ups and it's fun to flip giant tractor tyres but the whole idea behind CrossFit is to be as well-balanced as possible across all general skill areas, not just ones you're good at or enjoy the most. CrossFit is not about achieving specialised skills and fitness in one area. It is about achieving widespread physical ability.

***

Because I'm such a tight-arse with money, I made sure I got my money's worth from my unlimited one-month pass and attended as many CrossFit classes as humanly possible. I went every day for a month and after two weeks I was addicted. I forgot about getting bang for my buck and was thinking purely about my fitness. I could feel myself getting stronger and my mind had so much more clarity. I was hooked and when I was back from my work swing, I went twice a day, every day, where I could.

Around the same time, I travelled to Brisbane on my days off to compete in the 400 metre hurdles. It was my first serious race back after high school. It was nerve-wracking, but it was great to get back on the track. I felt really fit because I had been doing so many CrossFit sessions and I ended up placing first for my debut return. But that was to be the last competitive running race I ever took part in. I still continued my athletics but CrossFit was about to take over my life, and in a big way.

CHAPTER 7

Building Blocks

I signed up as a member at CrossFit Gladstone and officially became one of the converted. Other than Shane, I had no support network when I first moved to Gladstone so meeting like-minded people who enjoyed exercising and making friends was so refreshing. I looked forward to every morning and evening class. Training never felt like a chore.

"Back again, Tia? You can't get enough of it. Make sure you're not pushing your body too hard, you don't want to end up injuring yourself."

I could tell Sean was concerned that I was doing double sessions every day. It ticked me off though; I took it that he thought I wasn't up to it. I was like 'Man, who is this guy still telling me what to do. I'm coming in because I love the classes and they make me feel good.'

I went religiously for four months straight and not once did a competitive thought cross my mind. I didn't understand there were the CrossFit Games outside of regular classes or Regionals or anything like that. I just knew it was a really good fitness model and that it helped me with my overall fitness.

I was enjoying being competitive within myself and if I didn't like what I did in the morning then I could come back in the afternoon and try it all over again and beat my morning time! One afternoon,

I overheard the group of the fittest guys in the gym talking about a comp squad. It sounded like you had to be one of the best to be a part of it. It intrigued me, and I subconsciously started training with the comp squad at the back of my mind.

I got to the point where lots of people in the gym were telling me how strong I was and that I'd gone from strength to strength overnight. I felt it too and that maybe I could be good enough to be a part of the fit elite. But there was no way I was going to ask. I was way too stubborn and proud to do that. If I was ever going to be a part of something like that, the guys would have to ask me because I wanted them to want me and actually think I was good enough.

I waited for another couple of months and one day a guy by the name of Jake Knight asked me.

"Tia, we've got to pair up and start training for the next comp and I wanted to know if you want to join our squad and pair up with me?"

I felt the excitement surge through me but played it down to stay cool.

"Oh yeah, that would be fun, I guess. Thanks Jake, sounds good."

On the inside I was doing backflips. It was all I wanted, and I had earnt it.

Our first competition was on the Gold Coast, and I got paired with Jake. I didn't really know him well, but I knew he was an awesome CrossFit athlete. I thought to myself, 'Oh my God, you are paired up with a real athlete now so don't make any mistakes.' He was so passionate that he was yelling and screaming at me hard to motivate me.

I was crumbling in a pool of sweat, attempting to smash out my third round of 'King Kong'. If you struggle to lift heavy weights, then you have absolutely no chance in this workout. I had done my deadlift, two muscle-ups and squat cleans and I had my four handstand push-ups to go.

The squat cleans are always the hardest part for me. I had them out of the way which was good, but I was shaking.

"Unless you vomit, faint or die, keep going! Keep going, Tia! Push it harder, I know you can!"

It's a good thing I respond well to yelling because Jake was going hell for leather at me but boy, did it get my blood pumping! We trained flat out until the competition on the Gold Coast and I was so ready to compete.

Our other mates from CrossFit Gladstone had done their part and it was now up to Jake and me. We were placed fourth and we had to do two rounds of 15 deadlifts, 10 hang power cleans and 10 bar facing burpees.

"We've got to get in the top two. Just keep going, Tia, just keep going, don't stop to think about it! Don't feel the pain, there is no pain, just push through it!"

All I could hear was Jake yelling at me again, he wanted us to win so badly. I kicked into the zone and smashed out the rest of the set. We placed second and were stoked with our finish. I got a taste for being on the floor and I was hungry for more. CrossFit was meant to be just something I did for fun but after that comp, I fell madly in love with it.

I was enjoying CrossFit so much, I was more interested in training with others at CrossFit Gladstone than I was training by myself on the oval. It was a hard decision to make but halfway through 2013, after talking things through with Shane, I stopped competitive running altogether.

I did a couple more CrossFit team competitions and then made the big decision to sign up to my first individual CrossFit competition. I signed up a couple of months out and Shane and I made the plan to drive to Brisbane and compete in September 2013. I know Shane was so happy that I found something that gave me drive again and he was the first one to stand there and support me. We did classes together and he gave me pointers and feedback as he saw it. I needed extra training, as the general CrossFit classes weren't covering all the movements and there were movements coming up in competitions that I had never trained before. I was particularly nervous about legless rope climbs and strict handstand push-ups.

"Shane, the classes are great but I want to mix things up and break down more barriers. Maybe we could talk to Jake and get his thoughts on it all?"

We were cooling down and Shane took the opportunity to reach out to Jake for me.

"What the hell do we do here, mate? Tia is keen to step things up, but we don't have the faintest idea what we're doing."

"How about I show you what program I follow from my coach from up north and we'll go from there?"

Jake was so willing to help and shared everything he knew about the sport. Shane set up a gym for me in our garage at home, full of Rogue gear so we could do some of our programming there. I wanted to make sure that I did well at my first comp. I didn't want to embarrass Shane or my CrossFit gym.

Shane knew enough about weights and developing fitness because he always had a passion for strength and conditioning programs but only the basics. He understood the principles of a deadlift, squat, press and bench press; basically, all of the necessary movements people learn at a traditional gym but he wanted a second opinion.

In the early stages, Shane brought a lot of knowledge to the table but then we realised we needed more, especially when moves progressed over to gymnastics and Olympic weightlifting. Jake was a great friend during that time, he provided support and advice and worked out with me when he wasn't working.

"Shit, she's good, Shane. She really is good."

I overheard Jake giving me praise. He wasn't one to dish out compliments willy-nilly so I was pretty chuffed with myself. Jake's belief in me made me think I really could do well. I consider Jake a great friend and will always be thankful for him encouraging me to keep going.

***

I was in a rhythm with my training and I didn't worry about anything else other than committing to two sessions every single day, a CrossFit class and the workout Shane programmed for me. Once my training got serious, I started focusing on eating the right foods and getting proper sleep - which was challenging at times because of my shift work. My shifts were 12 hours, day and night, seven to seven, so I would go to the gym early, do the morning CrossFit class at 5 am, then go to work and come back in the night with Shane at 7:30 pm and train my program until 9 pm. It wasn't a chore; I just knew that if I trained hard, it would pay off. I don't necessarily love training, but I know it is fundamental to success and without it, I would have nothing. I know that I need to do it to do what I love most and that is compete.

"Shane, I am so exhausted, my muscles are sore and I don't feel like I'm improving. When I first started my numbers were always increasing. Now they have plateaued?"

"Trust in the process, babe, I can't believe how much you've improved just from your new program. If you keep this up, I honestly think you are capable of achieving anything."

Some days I would finish nightshift in the morning and go straight from work to the CrossFit morning class, where Nick or Jardan would coach me. After training I would go home and sleep, then come back to the gym to train before work that same night. There would be days where I would almost fall asleep at the wheel because I was so tired, but I would just keep pushing because I wanted to make the top 10 in my first individual competition.

There was one day where I had three night shifts in a row and on the Sunday, after already working Friday and Saturday nights, there was a little in-house competition that I really wanted to do in preparation for my competition in Brisbane. So, I did night shift, finished work, went to the competition, competed at CrossFit Gladstone and then went back and worked that night without any sleep. I was ruined.

Shane continued working with Jake on my programming and studied up on CrossFit and the Games every waking minute. I'm not kidding when I say he was consumed by it. Some days he would watch the CrossFit Games on the internet, other days he was glued to his iPad watching technique videos on YouTube or I'd walk into the office and he'd have 50 tabs open on his computer screen, reading the latest articles from the CrossFit Journal, crossfit.com or researching the most cutting-edge CrossFit equipment.

I didn't see the value in what Shane was doing at the time, but as the weeks crept up before the competition in Brisbane, Shane continued to surprise me with fantastic warm-up drills or strategies for different workouts. His self-education was helping big time.

CHAPTER 8

Hungry Again

Competition day arrived and far out, was I nervous. The comp was held at a local CrossFit box in Brisbane called CrossFit Cross-Axed. There were 40 people in the competition and I was hoping to finish in the top 10. The competition started on Friday night with one event because it was such a challenging workout they kept it by itself. It was a clean and jerk ladder but in between each lift, you had to do a round of 'Cindy' - five pull-ups, 10 push-ups and 15 air squats. My personal best was only 50 kilograms and the last barbell in the workout was 85 kilograms. Heading into the workout, Shane was trying to keep me focused and make sure I wasn't wasting energy thinking about the weight.

On paper and in my head, it seemed liked an impossible jump to achieve, mainly because I had never even attempted anything over 50 kilograms. I mentally stayed in the game and my spirits lifted every time I heard Shane, Jake and our friend Sam cheer me on in the crowd. I paced my way through each round of 'Cindy' and focused on nailing every clean and jerk, just like Shane and I had practiced.

I have no idea where the energy or the will came from, but I just kept pushing through. Every bar above 50 kilograms I kept telling myself 'Come on, Tia, you got this, the workout isn't over. Do it for

Shane, make the boys proud.' It was hard to not let the excitement overwhelm me, but I knew if I could just work my way through each bar one at a time and get as close as I could to the 85 kilograms, it would set me up well.

I was on the last bar of the event and I was the very first person to clear the entire ladder. At the end of the night I was coming third and said to myself, 'Holy shit, Tia this is your very first comp and you're coming third! Don't lose it now.' I managed to hold onto my spot over the next two days and made it to the finals. Just before I walked out on the floor, I headed to the girls' bathrooms and Shane grabbed me at the doorway.

"Now, Tia, you can do this. You just need to show them who you are and how hard you're willing to fight so they can't take this off you."

I listened to what he said and walked into the bathrooms. I looked in the mirror and stared at myself. I stood up tall and spoke out loud.

"You've got this, Tia."

I got my nervous wees out of the way and pulled myself together. Going into the finals, I thought I was coming first but I didn't know if it was by much. I knew there was only one option; I just had to go out there and give it hell. Jake had been there for the whole weekend, along with Shane and a couple of his best mates, Sam and Mousa. They were supporting me from the get-go and I didn't need anyone else. I was just super proud to have them in my corner, backing me to the end.

On the final day when the leaderboard showed me towards the top, it was crazy how many people who had brushed straight past me earlier in the comp like I didn't belong there suddenly showed interest in me. You could tell who was genuine and who wasn't. It was like they just wanted to jump in on the spotlight when I was showing signs of winning to show they were a part of our journey. It made me frustrated.

The atmosphere on the finals floor was penetrating and I was pumped. I looked around to embrace the environment but didn't take much notice of my competition because I was so focused on what I needed to do.

I only started training seriously in CrossFit two months earlier but I had trained my arse off. I felt strong, but I definitely wasn't experienced. Some of the women had been to Regionals prior to the event but that didn't bother me. If anything, it gave me more hunger to push harder and make my mark.

The final workout was three benchmark workouts put together – 'Fran', 'Grace' and 'Dianne' with a one-minute rest in between each and then I was done.

"Tia, I don't care where you are right now but you are going to show them why you deserve to be at the top."

I love hearing what Shane has to say, it always helps me refocus.

In my head I was thinking, 'So does that mean I'm coming first or second?' I didn't know where I was placed. I asked Shane, but he didn't tell me and out I went onto the floor. The countdown started three...two...one...and the PA beeped, the crowd erupted around us, people were yelling from every direction, it all compounded into one loud racket. I annihilated every workout and got further and further and further away.

The last bit of the finals was 'Dianne' and I had 21-15-9 reps of deadlifts and handstand push-ups. I was on the outside lane next to the crowd and I could hear Shane and the boys screaming so loud they were losing their voices. Even though there was no one else near me they just kept screaming because they wanted to see what I was capable of. Every rep, I felt the burn and wanted to stop but I could hear and feel their energy buzzing through me. 'Tia, you can't drop this bar otherwise they are going to get up you big time, push girl, push!'

I was motivating myself to push harder than ever before. The more I gained ground, the more go I had in me. I was feeding off myself. During my final reps, I looked over and saw the boys cheering me on and it gave me another surge of energy. I realised it was all or nothing. I finished my last set and dropped the bar down. 'I won, I fricken won!' I was speaking to myself over and over, I couldn't believe I actually won.

Other coaches looked confused; no one knew me or had even thought I was a threat. Before that moment, I really was a nobody. I looked over to my corner and Shane, Jake, Sam and Mousa were losing it. They looked like they were on one of those TV game shows and had just been told they're taking home a million dollars. They were jumping up and down, hugging each other with grins from ear to ear. I had done them proud. All of the time and effort they put into me paid off. I left no regret on the floor that day, there is no other feeling that compares to that.

I was so exhausted that I just wanted to fall in a heap and lay there for the rest of the night but I turned back around and cheered on the rest of the girls. It was more clapping and yelling because I was so breathless, but it was awesome to be a part of such a strong group of girls. Everyone finished their sets and came up to congratulate me, Shane and the boys made their way over too.

"Hell yeah, Tia, you did it!"

Jake was so ecstatic. I had never seen anything like it, he was hugging me and jumping around the place like he was on bloody Ecstasy. Shane gave me a big hug.

"I couldn't be prouder of you, T."

It was my first experience of individual competition in CrossFit and I loved it. I even won two thousand dollars in prize money. I took the time to sit down and chat with the other girls afterwards. It's one of my favourite things after a competition because at the end of the day, everyone goes through similar emotions and a similar training schedule as me. Sure, I may not know the girls on a personal level, but

I have a lot of respect for them because we share common experiences and are very like-minded people.

Shane and I were leaving the gym and one of the other coaches came up to me.

"Good work, Tia, who would have thought you'd do that well?"

His tone of voice was so condescending and I didn't understand why he was trying to have a dig at me. He kept standing there with his arms crossed.

"That's great that you did that but you have to remember that you haven't actually versed the best in Australia yet, so don't get ahead of yourself."

I saw red, I didn't understand why he was going out of his way to give me a backhanded compliment. I could feel my toes curl in my shoes and wanted to punch him square in the face.

'Don't retaliate Tia; he's just having a dig because his athletes didn't perform as good as what he wanted.' I was trying positive self-talk to myself so I didn't snap.

"Thanks for your kind words."

I forced a smile and walked away.

"Don't worry about him, babe, let's forget about that now. What he said is actually right but it's not for us to focus on right this minute. That doesn't matter and we don't care about that right now. One day we will verse the other girls and beat them but that's in the future, so just shut him out until we're ready."

Shane was right yet again and in a way, I should thank that random coach because that comment was one of those pivotal points in my life; where a naysayer said I couldn't do something and I took that negativity and turned it into ammunition to fire even harder.

Shane and I drove back up to Gladstone. We agreed that if I placed first in a competition that represents the majority of Queensland, then why wouldn't I give the Open a red-hot crack in 2014?!

CHAPTER 9
Miles

I was hungry to get better. I wanted to see how strong I could be if I dedicated more time to training. I enjoyed sessions with Jake, so we kept up our training whenever he got time off work - he always had a different program to follow which was good to get variety outside of the CrossFit classes. He often spoke about this weightlifting coach in Brisbane named Miles Wydall who was helping him with his technique. He sounded like the Godfather of weightlifting. I definitely needed help with my technique and, as it turned out, Miles had heard about me too and wanted to meet the young girl who clean and jerked 85 kilograms at only 54 kilograms in bodyweight. So, Jake reached out to him.

"I just got off the phone to Miles and he wants to meet you, Tia."
"What, really?!"

"He heard about your performance in Brisbane and wants to know more about you. When I told him you've only been doing CrossFit for a couple of months, he was even more impressed. He can't believe the numbers you hit."

Miles is a renowned Olympic weightlifting coach with over 20 years of experience in developing athletes from beginner to international representation. I couldn't believe that Miles, the guys I had heard so much about thought I was worth talking to. It was pretty surreal, but I needed all the help I could get if I was going to compete in the CrossFit Open so Shane and I drove six hours south to Brisbane.

*** * ***

We walked through the doors of the Cougars Weightlifting Club. The walls were covered in photos of famous Australian weightlifters and there on the floor in front of me were Commonwealth Games champion and two-time Olympian Damon Kelly and Commonwealth Games athlete Robert Galsworthy. Damon was doing back squats with an incredible amount of weight and Rob was doing snatches off the block at an unbelievable speed.

We sat down next to Miles and got chatting, and immediately I could tell how much Miles knew about this sport. He had an obvious passion for it and continued to reel off the weights of the guys' snatches, clean and jerks and squats. These athletes were heavy men, I mean like 105 kilograms plus and they were lifting five of me in weight. I was so inspired by the weight and speed they got under that bar, it blew my mind. It's not something I ever would have appreciated before and I know a lot of people don't, until you have to physically do it yourself.

"This is just so cool for me, Miles, I'm still not sure how I've ended up here and why I get to have the honour of watching an Olympic athlete train?"

"Well, Tia, with the numbers you produced at that competition, if you put the work in and develop your technique, you could possibly go to the 2016 Rio Olympics and the Commonwealth Games."

I felt like I had to clean my ears out. I couldn't believe what I was hearing, and Shane had that 'Are you kidding me?' expression glued to his face.

"From what I've heard, you've got hunger and natural ability, so all you need is to get more of an understanding of the sport and its technique and you can go to the Commonwealth Games and the Olympics."

Those words changed my life forever...

On the drive back home from Brisbane, I was still a bit taken back by what Miles had said but so excited to think I really had something big to train for. I asked Shane back-to-back questions the whole way home, rolling into my next question before he had a chance to answer my last question.

"Wow, those guys were amazing, I couldn't believe how much they were lifting."

"Miles is such a nice guy, he sure can talk the talk!"

"It's pretty crazy for him to say I could possibly make it to the Olympics, and he doesn't even know me, do you think he is just saying that?"

"He seems like a genuine guy, I don't think he would just that to anyone."

"Well, I guess we have some work to do."

Shane just started smiling to himself, I could tell he was so happy for me.

I always dreamed of going to the Olympics but never did I think I would try in weightlifting. I thought it would be for 800 metres but if I had the opportunity to go in a different sport I wasn't going to turn it down because it had always been a dream of mine. Plus, the area I needed to improve on the most with my CrossFit was strength and technique and weightlifting complemented this perfectly.

***

I owe a lot to Miles, he turned me from an amateur weightlifter into a professional athlete pretty much overnight and the craziest thing is that he wanted absolutely nothing from me. He didn't say I needed to choose between CrossFit and weightlifting; he supported me in doing both and wanted nothing more than to help me achieve. It was hard to believe that someone would care that much and put themselves out like that. We got into our training straight away. Shane and Miles worked together to ensure I had the best program tailored to my needs; Shane programmed my CrossFit training and Miles programmed my weightlifting. Shane would send Miles daily videos of me on his iPhone. Miles would write back with short simple feedback: 'straighter pull', 'bum down', 'wider grip.'

I smashed out a big legs session, Shane videoed my deadlifts and we sent it to Miles. My movements felt better than ever and I was looking forward to Miles' feedback. We got home and started cooking dinner; I couldn't believe how much my appetite was increasing from training. I was enjoying eating more food and I could feel myself getting stronger.

"Miles sent a reply to my video, Tia."

"Cool, what did he say!?"

"He said 'shoulders back'."

"Huh, is that it? What else did he say? Did he think it was good?"

"He's not there to blow smoke up your arse, babe, he's there to make you better."

Shane was right, and that reply summed up Miles in a nutshell. He's such a kind-hearted honest man, yet he is so technical and doesn't sugarcoat or overcomplicate anything. He just says it how it is and gets the job done. He understands the sport and what it takes to win like no one else.

The thing about Miles is he will go above and beyond with all of his athletes, whether they are Olympians or a middle-aged individual that does weightlifting as a hobby. He does like to set the ground rule that he will put in fifty per cent effort if the athlete puts in the other fifty per cent, but ask any of his athletes and they'll say he is generally the one putting in sixty per cent and the athlete forty per cent. There were times when I forgot to send him videos or reply to his messages, but he never flaked out on me. He always led the communication, keeping the momentum going and ensuring I was getting better. I followed this training program three days a week for 12 days in preparation for my competitions.

1.0 INTERMEDIATE GENERAL TRAINING PROGRAM

Power Snatch and Power Clean Jerk of **90%** off PB Snatch and Clean and Jerk, Snatch Squats off **110%** PB Snatch Squats off PB Front and Back Squats, Shoulder Press off PB Shoulder Press, Push Press off **80%** off PB Clean and Jerk, Snatch Pulls off **125%** of PB Snatch and Clean Pulls off **125%** RDL work off 90% Snatch or Clean.

WEEKS 1/3/5/7		
MON	**WED**	**FRI**
Snatch	Power Snatch	Power Clean Power Jerk
Power Clean Power Jerk	Clean and Jerk	Snatch
Front Squat	Back Squat	Front Squat
Clean Pulls	Snatch Pulls	Clean Pulls

WEEKS 2/4/6/8		
MON	**WED**	**FRI**
Clean and Jerk	Power Clean Power Jerk	Power Snatch
Power Snatch	Snatch	Clean and Jerk
Back Squat	Front Squat	Back Squat
Snatch Pulls	Clean Pulls	Snatch Pulls

WEEK 1/2/3/4	TECHNICAL	STRENGTH
	5/3 75%	4x5r 80%

WEEK 5/6/7	TECHNICAL	STRENGTH
	4/3 75%	3/5r 80% 2/3 85%

WEEK 8/9	TECHNICAL	STRENGTH
	5/2 80%	6/3r 85%

WEEK 10	TECHNICAL	STRENGTH
	Work to Max	4/2r 90%

WEEKS 11		
MON (light)	**TUE** (medium)	**FRI** (heavy)
Power Snatch	Power Snatch	Snatch
Power Clean Power Jerk	Power Clean and Jerk	Clean and Jerk
Snatch Pulls	Front Squats	Back Squats

WEEK 11	TECHNICAL	STRENGTH
Light	Work to 85% 1/1	3/2r 80%
Medium	Work up to 90% for 1	2/2 85% 2/1 90%
Heavy	Work up to Max for 1	5/1 90%

WEEK 12 – TAPER	
SESSION 1 (TUES)	**SESSION 2 (THURS) – SAT LIFT**
Snatch 2/2 80%, 1/2 , 85%	Power Snatch – 80% 3/2,
Clean and Jerk 2/2 80%, 1/2 , 85%	Power Clean and Power Jerk 80% 3/2,
Front Squat 3/2 off 90% C and Jerk,	Back Squat 3/2 off 90% Clean and Jerk,
Clean Pull 3/2 100% off PB Clean and Jerk	Snatch Pull 100% 3/2 off PB Snatch

I was developing strength at a rate of knots and lapping it up. I already had solid foundations in my lower body when it came to endurance-based workouts, but I was always very weak in the squat because I had never trained in a full-depth squat position. I worked morning and night to improve everything. I did squats, squats and more squats. I was obsessed with feeling the strain and pushing through the pain but one afternoon when I was training with the boys, I pushed too hard and felt something pop.

"Oh shit, something doesn't feel right! When I was coming up out of the squat, I felt something pop in my lower right side back."

I racked the bar back into the squat rack and then tried to stretch out my right side but there was still a dull ache. I finished the rest of my training off for that afternoon. My back got progressively worse, but I just kept telling myself to harden up.

Shane constantly checked in with me to see how it was and I kept telling him it was fine because I felt like I had come too far to stop now, and I really wanted to make Regionals and compete in the 2014 Glasgow Commonwealth Games trials.

Miles and Shane registered me in a couple of practice competitions leading into the trials which were in March on the Gold Coast. I didn't want to sacrifice the opportunity to compete, so I kept quiet about my back pain and insisted on training harder.

I kept going and I felt my lower back deteriorating. It became a constant ache and sometimes very sharp pains but that still wasn't stopping me. As my training progressed, Miles began educating Shane in weightlifting, teaching him everything he knew when it came to technique and the development of an athlete. It got to the point where Shane was taking things he had learnt from Miles and pulling together his own program for me, incorporating weightlifting and CrossFit training, which was much easier for me to follow.

I know I might be biased but I have the best coach in the world in Shane. When it comes to getting me mentally and physically prepared for CrossFit, weightlifting, running – absolutely anything really – he is second to none. He is willing to learn from anyone and everyone and not let ego get in the way. He spends hours on the computer doing his own research to expand his knowledge and if he doesn't know or understand something, he will be the first to reach out to others and ask their advice. I am so lucky that he is my partner as well as my trainer. He knows me innately and knows exactly what I'm feeling when I lift because he trains my program himself and does it with me.

I worked harder and harder with double days, which was exhausting alongside my nightshifts at work, but I needed as much training as I could get. I surprised myself at the Open, placing twentieth in Australia which put me in a good frame of mind going into the Commonwealth Games trials in March.

Miles supported me as my competition coach for weightlifting and Shane came along to help me warm up. The environment was quite intense, and I was on edge. My back was so sore, and it was my first major comp, so my emotions were running crazy. I started taking it out on Shane.

"Shut up, Shane, I don't want to do that weight, you don't understand how I'm feeling."

"Tia, I'm just trying to help you and do what we practiced."

Each time Shane said something, I bit back. I was being horrible and it was affecting my warm-up prep. My attitude made Miles uneasy; he was worried that I would bomb out on the platform and wasn't focused. Shane gave me one more piece of constructive feedback and I snapped back again.

"Tia, pull your fucking head in! We need you to focus on the task at hand and lift the bar. Shane and I will focus on everything else. You're up now, so pull your shit together and get out on that platform and lift the fucking bar."

I jumped out of my skin. I couldn't believe this well-respected, gentle, generous man came out and said that. I must have really overstepped the mark. Shane said nothing; he was probably just relieved Miles called me out.

I went out on that floor and started to lift. I was halfway through the comp and both Shane and Miles were crunching numbers together. I looked over at the guys deep in thought and it was at that moment that I realised how lucky I was. I knew I had the best team behind me. It was the very last lift of the comp and we were up to 101 kilograms but my personal best was only 85 kilograms so I was well out of my league.

"I want you to go out there on 101 kilograms and rip that bar off the ground. Just get on in there and rip it!"

Miles shook me with passion and I felt it run through me.

"You just have to go out there and do it because I know you can do it.'

"If you hit this lift there's a possibility you could get selected for the 2014 Glasgow Commonwealth Games."

I couldn't believe what Miles just said and Shane got right behind him.

"Come on, babe, go get it!"

I was shitting bricks, Shane and Miles were both backing me. I felt the adrenaline building in my body ready to explode, thinking to myself, 'I could die under this much weight'.

I walked out onto the floor, took a big breath and I cleaned it. I fucking cleaned it off the ground! It wasn't pretty, I had to squeeze out of the bottom, grunting, but I cleaned it and got the bar up. I paused in the front rack position for what felt like eternity but celebrated too early and lost the jerk in front of me. But it didn't matter. Shane and Miles were smiling brighter than the sun. The fact that I had pulled my shit together, gone out there and just cleaned it right off the floor was crazy. It is one of the highlights of my athletic career and was the turning point of me believing that I can do whatever I set my mind to. I was only 56 kilograms and I had only been weightlifting for a couple of months, but I walked out on that floor and cleaned almost twice my body weight. I was so proud.

World class weightlifters and men and women from famous weightlifting families were coming up to me and congratulating me. I kept hearing 'You're going to be good, Tia, you're going to make it.' For people to say that after one lift that I actually failed gave me the assurance that I was choosing the right path.

That day was a total wake-up call. I realised that I wasn't the only one on this journey. So many people close to me were by my side, willing to sacrifice everything in order me for me to achieve my goals. It was that day that I knew I had to repay Shane and Miles for their commitment to me by working hard and making it to the 2016 Rio Olympics.

CHAPTER 10

Setbacks

I made the shadow team for the Commonwealth Games. I was a bit upset I didn't qualify but I also didn't expect to get as far as I did, so I didn't stew on it for long. Competing at the Commonwealth Games trials was thrilling and to experience being that close yet not really taking it seriously made me want to go to the Olympics even more. I had no plans to podium at the Olympics but I wanted to be a part of it, so I said to myself, 'You've got two years to qualify for the Olympics, give it your everything and then you can live with yourself and move on with your life, knowing you did everything possible.'

I told Shane my goal was to go to the CrossFit Games and the Olympics in the same year. He was supportive but when I told some of my other close family and friends they thought I was too ambitious. It didn't bother me what they said or thought, I believed in my ability. I was highly motivated and wanted to put in the work to get there but I felt like I couldn't give one hundred per cent because of my back.

I still didn't really know what the problem was, but I had to keep training because the CrossFit Regionals were only two months after the Commonwealth Games trials. My main focus was getting to Regionals, giving it my best shot and just seeing where I ranked. I didn't have any ambition to go to the Games that year but I was keen to see what all the hype was about at Regionals. I travelled to

Wollongong in May 2014, where 30 athletes from Australia and New Zealand and 10 athletes from Asia met to compete with only the top three going through to the Games.

I worked hard on all the moves and events that were released two weeks earlier. Shane and I trained with the goal of completing every event and placing in the top 15. One of the workouts incorporated a legless rope climb which I had never done before, so when the workout got released I practiced it, maybe even over-practiced it, and felt confident going into Regionals. But it was a disaster. I went out too hard and burnt out in the fourth round, completing the workout unsuccessfully. I could hear Shane and Jake yelling at me to shake out the arms and my friends that travelled down from CrossFit Gladstone were cheering me on to keep going but I had nothing left and kept failing the climb. I walked over to Shane after the workout and fell into him, crying.

"How did I go from being able to do that in training to not even being able to progress to the halfway mark?"

"Tia, you've tried your hardest, babe. There's nothing else you could have done. Don't look at this as a failure, look at this as a learning curve and next time we'll be stronger and better. We're going to learn from this. I want you to give it your best for the rest of the day."

There were more tears than talking because I didn't want to hear anything, I just wanted comfort. I was so disappointed in myself. The event wasn't at all what I thought it was going to be and the negative experience turned me off CrossFit for the rest of the year.

More than most, I can appreciate that in a competitive environment, people aren't there to make mates, they are there to win. However, I believe there's a fine line between being professional and being rude. Regionals 2014 didn't match my expectations. In the lead-up, I had heard so much great stuff about the event's comradery and buzzing atmosphere but there was none of that.

It became evident early on that the athletes were clearly divided into two groups – the veteran CrossFit athletes and the new CrossFit rookies, who were yet to be paid the respect from the professional athletes. Shane shrugged it off but it just didn't sit right with me. I felt like everyone who was there deserved it and deserved to be respected. Feeling like an outsider was horrible and is something I will always take into consideration now that the shoe is on the other foot. I would never want other aspiring CrossFit athletes to feel the way I did that day and will never look past a rookie. I will make sure they're having fun and feeling comfortable because after that experience I was willing to give up everything. I wasn't going to do it if it wasn't enjoyable.

One of the final workouts at Regionals consisted of handstand push-ups, front squats and burpees and I couldn't even walk off the floor, I was in so much pain. I hobbled off because I couldn't stand up straight. Once I told Shane about how bad my back really was, he was mad and told me I was to have four months off completely. What a blow, I felt like crap.

I went to get x-rays and MRIs which showed a fractured spine. It definitely isn't the worst injury but boy, it was painful. There was bleeding inside the bone because of damage to the bone marrow from jarring it so many times. I had put so much stress on my back that the bone started to develop fractures. The only solution was rest.

I was completely deflated and so angry with myself that I let something that could have been easily treated get so bad. I just had to accept it because it was out of my own stupidity that my injury got to that point. I failed to look at the bigger picture. I was focused on Regionals in such a short-term way and paid the price of doing what turned out to be six months of nothing.

***

In July 2014, Shane and I were all booked and ready for Vegas! We decided to go overseas with our friends, KB and Travis, to celebrate my twenty-first birthday. Everyone was keen to go to the CrossFit Games in Carson, California on the back end of our trip.

"Guys, that's stupid. There are so many other things to do, let's not waste our time sitting in a stadium. The only time I ever want to go to the Games is as a competitor."

"Stop being such a spoilsport, Tia. I bet you'll like it when we go there, and besides, you can see what those athletes actually go through."

"Pffft, I'm done with it, Shane."

Even though I'm no party animal, I still loved being in Vegas with my friends and once we were over there, I was a little more excited about the prospect of going to the Games and when the boys saw that I was warming to the idea, they went ahead and booked.

"I know I need to stop being so bitter and I will, I've just never imagined being in this situation, that's all. One thing I am looking forward to now, is seeing Denae Brown compete, I just love her."

I saw Denae at Regionals and she was incredible. She had just had a baby and bounced back to win the Regionals after one year away from competition. I was in awe of her and thought if anything, at least I can go and cheer her on. We went along and started watching every individual event and I think I was the one who ended up enjoying it the most. I was so proud to be Australian and to see the girls compete at that level.

"Wow, Shane, look at them all go, they really deserve to be there."

"We can get there too, Tia, I honestly think we can do it. It would take complete commitment but you're just as talented as these women."

Shane doesn't say those things unless he believes it to be true so I definitely took notice of it, even if I didn't show it.

Attending the 2014 Games as a spectator was a humbling experience and made me really appreciate the calibre of athletes. There was one moment in particularly when Camille Leblanc-Bazinet was announced as the winner and she and her husband had a special moment on the floor. The satisfaction I saw on Camille's face when her husband came over and hugged her filled my heart completely. I could see that they had gone through so much together and that they had finally gotten their reward. I sat back and had tears of joy. I was so happy for them and hoped I could share something like that with Shane one day.

We travelled some more, then got home to Gladstone. I hadn't exercised in four months; I put on weight and felt lethargic all the time. The pain was slowly disappearing, I just had to make sure I was standing upright or laying down flat. When I made a sudden movement, I could still feel a little bit of pain through my spine but it was definitely on the up.

I was the heaviest I've ever been. I weighed 63 kilograms which was shocking for me because I was always used to weighing 56 kilograms and for a small person, seven kilograms is a lot of weight. Seeing Shane still go and exercise was really frustrating too, because all I wanted was to go to the Olympics and I felt like I was running out of time. The five months finally came around and in November 2014, I started to move. I couldn't really feel the pain anymore so I went for walks and did my low impact rehab exercises. I wasn't allowed to do any high intensity or anything that involved picking up objects. I did Pilates and movement pattern drills for a month to activate my inner core but the hardest thing was starting to pick up the barbell. In December 2014, I returned to my first CrossFit class. Even though I had written it off after Regionals, I still decided to do the classes because I truly believed in the CrossFit training methodology and knew it would help my weightlifting.

CHAPTER 11

Our Box

During rehab, I enjoyed Pilates the most because I was progressing and moving in the right direction but as soon as I picked up the bar and couldn't do what I used to be able to, that's when it hurt - my spirit more than my body. At first, we did light weights at home. I wasn't myself, I was overcautious and over-communicating, telling Shane about every little niggle or concern I had, to the point where we were doing more talking than training.

Shane had been so supportive with my recovery but I was so up and down all the time that I could see his patience wearing thin.

"Babe, I don't need to hear about every little niggle you think you might have, it's not adding any value. I know you're worried about hurting yourself again but come on, Tia, let's get ballsy and have a real crack."

My mate Travy came along to one of my sessions with me and could see it too.

"You're not injured anymore, Tia, you need to get out of your own head. Don't over-think, just listen to your body and take action."

I couldn't snap out of it, I kept looking for pain and bailed out early on all of my movements. I'd be in an overhead squat and would have tears streaming down my face. I was so confused as to whether it was a good or a bad pain and didn't understand my body properly. Two weeks passed and Shane took action.

"Miles is coming up for a few days to go over some technique training with you. He'll take you back to basics and let's see if that gets you back in your groove."

I was so grateful to Shane for sticking it out with me and felt relieved to see Miles. Miles cut through everything and made me feel safe in my movements so it started feeling normal again.

"I don't know what you're so worried about. You're on the right track, just keep building like that and you'll be good to go. I'm not worried at all."

The reassurance was all I needed. I built myself up and continued to remind myself of what Dad would always say. 'Just take it day by day; don't think about a month, next week or next year. Think about the now and focus on what are you doing right now to make yourself better.'

I eased back into my training and made sure I was doing absolutely everything to get back to where I was before I was injured and the more I put in place, the more I trusted the process. Each time I felt shitty or like I was running out of time in my training week or not hitting PBs, I asked myself, 'Have you put one hundred and ten percent into every single training session? Yes. Have you gone over your nutrition and ensured it's flawless? Yes. Have you made sure your recovery is up to scratch and you're tapping into all of the resources and equipment available to you? Yes.'

I put things in place to ensure the answer was always 'yes'. Having that confidence in myself helped me back my own abilities. I knew there was nothing else I could be doing and that everything would be okay because of all my hard work.

At the end of the day, it didn't matter what recovery program I was on or what my surroundings were. It came down to the simple fact that I really wanted to get to the Olympics and I was willing to push myself outside of my boundaries, to get back to where I left off. Not only did I get back to my original state but improved in all aspects of my training.

***

I became much smarter and more in tune with my body. I listened to the warning signs and communicated with Shane when I felt a niggle. If my wrist started to hurt, we avoided exercises and movements that engaged it. Then as soon as I got home at night, I made it my number one priority to focus on loosening my muscles and doing everything to make it better for the next day.

Not once did I stop my training altogether. I began resting the right parts of my body or having two rest days instead of one, making simple adjustments to ensure I was still getting better whilst not overdoing it.

Recovery became a critical part of my schedule. I got massages, did sauna sessions, used my NormaTec boots at night and rolled out on my foam roller and lacrosse ball.

On Christmas Day, I spoke to Mum and Dad about quitting my job and putting everything into making the Olympics.

"I'm never going to have another opportunity like this so I think I need to leave my job. I know it's a great paying job and everything but I can't commit to my training with the shift work."

"We'll support you, T, but you need an income of some sort."

"I'm going to see if I can work for CrossFit Gladstone, it seems like the obvious option and Shane is happy for me to do that too."

It was a hard decision to make and it took some time for me to actually hand in my resignation letter at work, but when I did I felt so much relief.

I was at CrossFit every day from 4 am until 9 pm and my love for training was reignited, not that I ever lost it. I was just so let down by Regionals the year before and it left a bad taste in my mouth. The taste slowly disappeared and my love for CrossFit got deeper the more I coached people and became part of their fitness journey, it was awesome. It's so true that every box is its own family and the family at CrossFit Gladstone meant a lot to me. Watching everyone come together before a training session was like walking into a big family barbeque where the room is buzzing with love and laughter.

As I was making the transition from Rio Tinto to CrossFit Gladstone, Benito told me he was ready to sell his share of the gym and asked if I was interested in buying it. I was only 21 and it was a big move for someone so young who had no business experience, but I needed an income to support my new CrossFit and weightlifting career. My parents gave me the good conservative advice that it's a bad idea going into business with someone else and that it probably wasn't a smart move, given I wanted to focus on my own training. But I decided to go ahead with it.

The challenge excited me and Shane said he would back me so I became a business owner. I had a business partner who lived an hour and a half away and wasn't very involved with the gym so I had to really rely on Jardan, my gym manager, to help me understand the procedures of the gym. The gym was running at a loss and I needed to make some serious changes otherwise there wasn't going to be a CrossFit Gladstone anymore. I tightened up on our outgoings and wages. We had 15 staff on the books which wasn't sustainable. I wanted everyone to stay on as a coach so I decided the most cost-effective way was to give the coaches a free membership in exchange for coaching a couple of classes a week.

The first six months of owning CrossFit Gladstone was a very challenging time for me, I had to make big decisions to keep the business afloat which didn't suit everyone. However, if it wasn't for being decisive and making those decisions, our box wouldn't be there today. I don't think I would have done as well as I have in my athletic career without that experience because that period in my life was character-defining and made me stronger and more resilient. I learnt to stand my ground and not let the hard times get me down. Any challenging moments in my life I like to take head-on, and convert any feelings of hurt and anger into drive and determination to achieve even more.

CHAPTER 12

Game On

I was at the point where all I wanted to do was get strong for weightlifting. My programming focused on doing lots of isolated movements, banded work and accessory training to strengthen my lower back. My long-term goal of making the Olympics in 18 months was my only focus. I was doing double training days and was so consumed by my program that the CrossFit Open came around before I knew it.

"Open is here!"

Shane was bouncing around the kitchen getting excited about the first week of the Open. I got the sense that he was trying to get me up and about for it too.

"You may as well give it a proper shot, hey babe, and see how far you get?!"

Even though I said I never wanted to compete for CrossFit again, Shane knew me well enough to know I only said that out of anger. As a CrossFit affiliate owner, I wanted to participate in the Open for my members, so I committed to taking part. By the time week three of the Open came around, something inside me fired up. I was halfway through fifteen point three and was smashing through my wall-balls. Something clicked during the workout, it's like I wasn't even fatigued and just kept going faster and faster. The timer beeped and I slammed my ball to the floor. I was surprised by my own ability and smashed out the final week, coming seventh in Australia.

It was a great result, especially given where we'd come from and that our focus had been on weightlifting and running our gym, not competing for the Games. Shane and I packed up the gym after everyone went home, walked over to our car at the back of the gym and put our bags in the boot.

"Shane, I'm going to make the CrossFit Games."

I was so adamant, there was a long pause and Shane just looked me.

"I'm going to the CrossFit Games, Shane!"

I don't know where it came from or why I said it. But it just made sense. I had everything there in front of me in order to succeed. I left my job, owned a gym and had access to all of the equipment. It was set up perfectly, so why not do it?

"Well okay, Tia, but we're really going to have to pick up the work then, it's just around the corner."

"I know, I'm going to do it."

As a coach myself, I hear people say all the time, 'I'm going to go to the Games'. And I always say, 'That's awesome, why do you want to go to the Games?' and I go through all of the commitments and sacrifices with them. So, when I make a statement like that, I know how outrageous it is and how much it takes, so I would never say it if I didn't mean it.

"Right, Tia. Tomorrow, we start".

We only had three months to get me to where I needed to be. It was no easy feat. In previous years, the top 30 athletes from the Open qualified for Regionals and the top three athletes from Regionals qualified for the Games. But for the first time in 2015, it was the top five athletes that qualified for the Games. So I set my own goal of placing in the top three just so I knew that even if the new rules weren't in place, I still would have made it to the Games. I didn't want to settle for four or five.

Shane upped my sessions from two to three a day. We did triple days because we were so far behind. We also figured the Games are three full-day competitions anyway so I should train as I would compete. There was a lot of volume in each day and we structured our days to reflect the Games. The only difference was my average weekly training output was always around eighty per cent of my full capacity, with some workouts at sixty per cent and other workouts at one hundred per cent Shane would say, 'Okay, this workout is all about max effort,' or 'I want you to back off intensity and focus on technique.' He is great at keeping things interesting so he'd get me to see how many muscle ups I could do in three minutes or go for a 14-minute run and tell me to forget about meeting a certain time and focus on cruising naturally, doing what I love.

Going into the 2015 Regionals, I had no emotion. I was solely focused on qualifying for the Games and not letting any of the other girls affect me this time around. I walked into the stadium and said hello to the people that acknowledged me but didn't let the raw emotions of other athletes get to me.

No one knew who I was, only the people I had met from the previous year. I continually reaffirmed my ability from the moment I walked through those stadium doors, 'Tia, just enjoy it and do the complete opposite to last year. You're so strong and so capable.'

It was the last event of the Regionals and I had completed 10 of my 15 muscle ups. Kara Webb was in front of me and I was chasing her tail. My body was sore from the weekend's work but I knew if I gave up, the disappointment I'd feel afterwards would be nothing compared to the physical pain I was feeling now. 'You play your game; you stick to the strategy Shane gave you.' I gathered and composed myself. I overdid it a bit in my muscle ups but I got there in the end and smashed out my clean ladder. I nearly tripped over the bar when I crossed the finish line but I made it and I took the podium in third place.

The feeling of standing on those blocks and qualifying for the Games after all the shit I had been through, was indescribable. I wanted to put CrossFit Gladstone on the map and I did. All I could think about was my members and mates who had stuck by me. I did it for them. I know it's biased but I am so proud of how far our gym has come. I could not be happier, the members we have are incredible, they turn up to have fun, get fit and be part of all the positive vibes, it's the best atmosphere to be a part of.

***

I had only been doing CrossFit classes for two years and was still so new to it all. It was a huge shock to get to the Games in California, let alone place second and take home eighty thousand dollars in prize money. I couldn't believe I got paid for doing something I loved. I didn't even know we got paid for placing, so that was just a cherry on top when I found out.

Shane and I arrived in Carson and it was buzzing with fifty thousand people all awaiting the 2015 CrossFit Games and this time I was a competitor. The heat on the first day was so intense, it was uncomfortable to be outside for longer than five minutes so it was great to start the Games in the water with the Pier Paddle. Swimming is my strength, so placing fourth in my first event gave me the start I needed. Most of the 2015 Games feels like a blur to me. The only workout I seem to really remember is 'Murph'. It was the first time a hero workout was included in the Games and involves a 1-mile run, 100 pull-ups, 200 push-ups, 300 squats and another 1-mile run, while wearing a weighted vest of 14 pounds.

We all lined up and I could hear the other girls commenting on how hot and humid it was. I could feel it as well but it didn't feel too different to where I grew up in Weipa. Halfway through the event, athletes started pulling out because of the heat. A couple of the girls suffered heat strokes and some even pulled out of the Games all together. I finished in twenty-seventh place. It was tough going but that event has stuck with me, because it's when I realised the Games definitely isn't for the faint hearted.

The last day came around and I didn't know I had placed second overall until Andreas Gloor, the Marketing Manager from Reebok came up to me.

"Tia, do you know where you came?"

I had actually thought I had come fifth and was a bit disappointed because heading into the final event, I was sitting fourth and just wanted to hold my position.

"You placed second, Tia you're the second Fittest Woman on Earth!"

It was a massive surprise and completely unexpected because all I really wanted to do was not come last. When Andreas confirmed I came second, all I wanted to do was see Shane and my friends.

'The majority of the athletes didn't know me so I felt like everyone thought I didn't deserve to place second because a number of the well-known athletes couldn't compete to their full potential due to the heat stroke from Murph.' But I didn't care because as far as I was concerned, I had worked so hard to be there just like everyone else. Some of the other Aussie athletes came over to me cheering and jumping with excitement. It was such an incredible feeling because I was the first ever Australian to podium at the CrossFit Games.

I ran over to Shane and the surprise on his face was priceless, he was just so happy for me and all of our friends were so excited.

When Shane and I eventually got around to watching the 2015 Games highlights reel, I was a bit disappointed because I wasn't featured once. But in all honesty, no one knew who I was and it was a total shock placing second, some even said that it was a fluke. Even though I knew I worked hard and deserved to be there, it did play on my mind a bit. I would ask myself, 'Was it a fluke and did I only podium because other people pulled out or couldn't perform to their best?" For such a high point in my life, it put a bit of a dampener on for me. But the comment that got me the most was when I heard someone say in an interview, 'If I was Tia, I would be focusing on getting back to the Games and placing in the top 20." I was furious. I couldn't believe it; I had another person out there doubting my abilities so publicly. I never forgot that and kept those words in the back of my mind during my training. I wanted to show the whole world that it was no fluke.

CHAPTER 13
Strong is Sexy

Before CrossFit I always had a small muscular build and weighed about 52 kilograms. My muscle was predominately on my legs because of all the kilometres I ran growing up. When I first started CrossFit training, my muscle built up very quickly. It grew even more when I started training with Miles, especially when he got me to eat larger food portions to fuel my body. I developed a lot more strength but one thing I hadn't prepared myself for was the big changes in my appearance.

The biggest changes were in my arms and traps. I really filled out and bulked up, but I didn't realise how big I was until a month before we left for the 2015 CrossFit Games. I got ready to head out to dinner with Shane to our favourite Thai restaurant in town. When Shane and I go out, I love putting effort in and doing my hair and makeup so I can look nice for him and get out of my usual training clothes. I pulled my favourite strappy summer dress out of my wardrobe and put it on. It looked terrible, I was horrified. It was the first time I had looked at myself properly in the mirror without training clothes on and I looked like a boy. Shane heard me crying and came into the bathroom.

"What's wrong, Tia, you okay?"

"Look at this dress. The straps are meant to be loose and long and they're tight and the dress is sitting all funny on me. If this loose dress doesn't fit me, nothing will."

I was embarrassed and worried that Shane wouldn't find me sexy if I kept building more muscle. I got changed back into my training clothes and we went out for dinner. I was looking at all of the other girls at the restaurant in their little shorts and girly dresses and they all had such small frames, I started to envy them in a way.

"Tia, I think you are so beautiful and love you however you are. Building muscle is part of getting stronger and when you build muscle it's a permanent reminder to people of how strong you are. I think it's a great thing."

I felt a little bit better after Shane reassured me, but I was still miserable when it came to shopping.

"Let's go to the shops in Rockhampton and do some shopping, hey T?"

"I don't want to go, I won't be able to buy anything."

Shane made me go anyway and I ended up buying a new wardrobe of clothes that hid my muscles, especially my traps.

"Shane, it just makes me not want to get any bigger."

"Well, do you want to get stronger?"

"Yes."

"Well, that means you need to get bigger too and if you want to do this, then that's the path you've got to go down."

I knew he was right and I felt pathetic being so vain but it was hard to get used to.

"Just look at it like this Tia, ten years of your life is nothing. You can build the muscle and strength you require, then you go back to normal and fit back into your old-sized clothes. For now, you have to accept it because there is a bigger picture."

"Yeah, I know, it just sucks."

"Tia, let's be honest. Being able to fit into a dress isn't as important as going to the Olympics."

After I podiumed at the 2015 CrossFit Games and experienced being in a room with other amazingly beautiful and strong women, I finally realised how stupid I was being. I noticed myself admiring all of the other ladies' bodies and hearing other people comment on how strong and amazing everyone looked. I got flooded with the biggest sense of pride and felt empowered that I was a strong woman as well. I had the realisation that if I wanted to compete and make the Olympics that I needed to develop more strength.

The more I trained and the more I ate, the bigger I got. And the bigger I got, the more I started to notice my form getting better. Every time Shane and I would go out, he would compliment me and tell me things looked good. That's all I needed. My confidence grew and I really started feeling more comfortable with my body. I thought, 'Well, if Shane thinks I look good that's all that matters.'

I was so conservative that I used to wear bike pants and baggy long pants over the top and I wouldn't even wear three quarter leggings that were tight because I thought they showed too much bum. Once I had that boost of confidence, I started training in bummies and lots of the women at CrossFit Gladstone complimented me and said how great I looked. It felt good to hear people say nice things about my muscles and it was a real lesson for me to embrace who I am and what I look like and to celebrate my uniqueness.

***

I wish I'd liked my muscles from the get-go because now I love them and am so proud of them. I know there are millions of other women out there who are proud of their strong physiques and so they should be. I also know a lot of women cop constant criticism about not looking feminine or girly enough, which is absolute rubbish.

When ladies first start CrossFit, most of the time the first thing they say is 'I really don't want to get man arms and bulky legs.' I completely respect and understand that some women don't want to build muscle and prefer to focus on getting fit or losing weight. But sadly, I also think that those comments are a reflection of how society and the media tells women they should look and they're worried they won't conform if they get too muscular.

I know that's what I initially thought. Imagine if being muscular was the norm and popular culture promoted muscular women in lingerie campaigns. I bet fewer women would be making those comments and more would be keen to get strong and build muscle.

Every man and woman has the right to look however they want to look and people need to embrace that. The real issue is the pictures and information people are fed in the mainstream media depicting what femininity should look like. It's true that we don't really see many muscular women and when we do, stronger, more athletic female bodies often receive awful reactions.

In my eyes, there is nothing unusual about a muscular woman. What is unacceptable is women feeling like they can't reach their full physical and athletic potential because of the so-called rules of femininity. And that's what it came down to for me. I thought, 'Like hell am I sacrificing my dream of going to the CrossFit Games just so I can have thin arms and legs'. That was such a small, vain and unimportant factor in the big picture of achieving my dream. There was a point early on where my image did affect me but having the love and support of my family and friends put everything into perspective. When I train and use my body, just like Shane or any other guy, I become muscular and strong too. I want other women to feel empowered to train and use their bodies and not feel like they have to operate within a confined area. There is definitely a more recent shift in the media away from extreme thinness to more athletic figures but many women are still consumed by diet plans and weight loss and the fear of getting too muscular.

If there's one thing I'd like to see change, it's getting society to start thinking differently about muscular women. Women who exercise, train hard and keep their bodies healthy and fit are strong and capable and the world needs more of them.

CHAPTER 14

Olympic Qualifiers

The day after the 2015 CrossFit Games I said goodbye to Carson and set my sights on making the Australian Olympic weightlifting team for Rio 2016. I had tough competition and there was only one spot available across all the categories. There are one to two spots available across each of the weight categories for the Commonwealth Games but for the Olympics, only one Australian out of all of the weight categories qualifies so it's even more competitive. The Sinclair Equation helps determine which athlete qualifies. The Sinclair Coefficients are derived statistically and are adjusted each Olympic year. They are based on the Total World Records in the various bodyweight categories as of the previous several years. The formula to determine the strongest athlete is Actual Total x Sinclair Coefficient = Sinclair Total.

The first qualifying event for the Olympics was in Houston in November 2015 at the World Championships for weightlifting. It was one of three trials for the Olympics and I performed well, considering where I was ranked in the sport. I had two more opportunities after that and the next one was in December in Brisbane, directly after the CrossFit Invitationals in Madrid. It felt like I was constantly on the road but I was enjoying every minute of it.

Shane and I never fly Business Class. We will one day, but for now I would prefer to spend money on other things. Our seats on the flight back to Australia seemed particularly cramped so I got up every hour and followed my stretching routine at the back of the plane. I did 20 squats, 30 hip thrusts, hamstring stretches and shoulder rotations. I drunk water every hour to flush out the toxins and tried to sleep in between. I couldn't eat much either as I had to make sure my weight was down because of the fluid retention from flying.

Shane and I landed on Australian soil a day before the second weightlifting trial which wasn't ideal. The judges let me compete as a guest in another weight group so I could have one rest day before I lifted in my 58 kilograms category. Having to fly from Houston to Spain and back to Australia, competing at every destination was taxing, to say the least. I was physically exhausted, sore and jetlagged.

I started my warm up with Miles and Shane and we went through the usual dynamic movements to get my body ready. I kept catching the eyes of a group of coaches standing in front of me. After a while it became obvious that they were talking about me. They were standing directly in my eye line, whispering in each other's ears, trying to put me off. Shane must have seen me getting a little frazzled.

"Don't worry, I can see what they're doing, Tia. They're trying to play games from a distance. Just ignore them."

Miles, came right in behind Shane and backed me up.

"Tia, they're trying to get to you and they can't. I want you to go out there and lift like you've never lifted before and when you do it, look through them like they're invisible. They can't do anything to screw you over. It comes down to which athlete can produce the best result and I know you won't give up easily."

I walked out onto the floor and went for it. I hit my target weight 83 kilograms snatch and 111 kilograms clean and jerk. Miles ran over to me and hit my back a lot harder than I think he meant to and winded me a little but he couldn't help it, he was so pumped.

"AWESOME, Tia. Good job! That's exactly what we needed."

Miles was always so composed and it was so great to see him show so much emotion. I knew I had made him proud.

I hit my target but it wasn't officially over. Miles and Shane were just so excited because I put up such a big total that everyone was now chasing me. I wanted the spot badly and fought for it hard because I knew it could be my only opportunity to get to the Olympics. Everything was happening so quickly and I had one more trial to perform at in Fiji before I knew if I qualified.

There is a lot of jealousy in the weightlifting world from other coaches because I compete in the CrossFit Games. After that event, a few coaches made comments that I did not deserve to go to the Olympics because I competed in the Games and wasn't solely focused on weightlifting.

One of the coaches came up to me at the end of the competition and had a dig.

"In the rule book, it says an athlete must be solely focused on weightlifting to be selected for the Olympics. What do you have to say about that?"

I wanted to say, 'Stop being such a sore loser,' but I wouldn't dream of dropping to his level.

"I work really hard and I know I deserve it."

I responded politely and walked away. It was frustrating because the last thing I was doing was taking weightlifting for granted. I was training so hard for the sport, if not harder than most. I didn't raise it with anyone because I felt like I always had the support from the Australian Weightlifting Federation and that's all that mattered. So I said nothing and killed them with kindness. I just had to get that Olympic spot and let my ability do the talking.

Miles told me that some of the coaches came up to him and complained as well.

"I said to them, Tia, if they've got a problem, then all they need to do is beat you in Fiji. They didn't have too much to say to that."

I loved Miles, he always had my back and kept shit real.

It was so satisfying placing first, knowing I had still done everything in the lead up and didn't have to say no to other events and competitions. I know sometimes I won't be able to do everything but I don't want to say no to things out of fear. I wasn't willing to give up going to the CrossFit Invitationals out of fear that I wouldn't win the trials because I thought, 'What happens if I don't make the Olympics and I missed such an awesome life experience at the Invitationals?' I truly believe that in order for me to be successful, I need to enjoy my journey and what that means for me is doing whatever I want throughout my career to make me happy. And if I'm happy, I can guarantee myself that I will be successful. The only time I won't be successful is if I lose sight of my number one priority. My only priority in 2015 was to go to the CrossFit games. In 2016, my priorities were to place second or better at the CrossFit Games and go to the Olympics and they came at different stages of the year, so I was able to prioritise them accordingly.

What I'm trying to say is that there is a time and a place for priorities. A lot of athletes will refuse to go on certain trips or experience certain things as they fixate on one particular thing. I know that everyone's process is different, just like everyone's training program is different, but for me that's not a well-rounded life. Living in that way doesn't make me happy and if I'm not happy, I can't achieve. I want to look back on my career and have no regrets because I experienced everything.

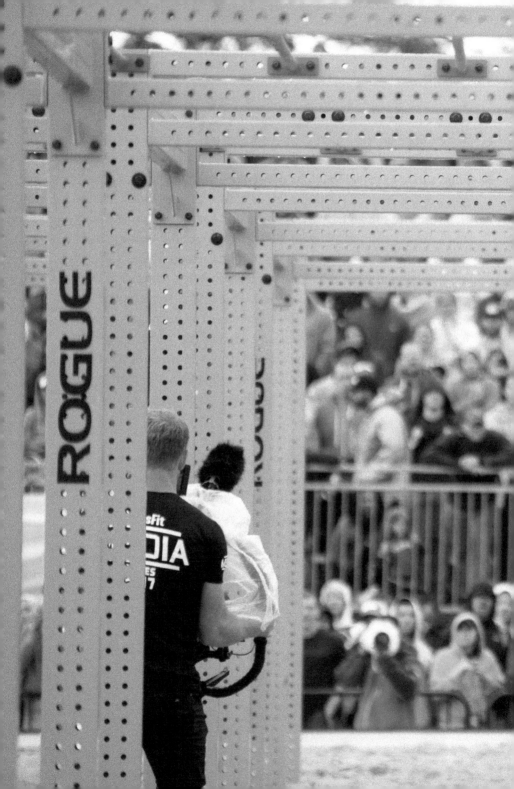

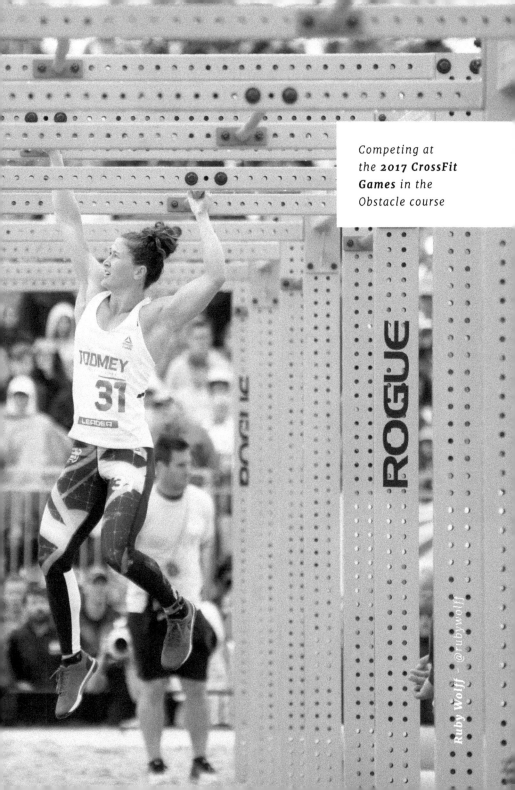

Competing at the *2017 CrossFit Games* in the Obstacle course

Ruby Wolff ~ @rubywolff

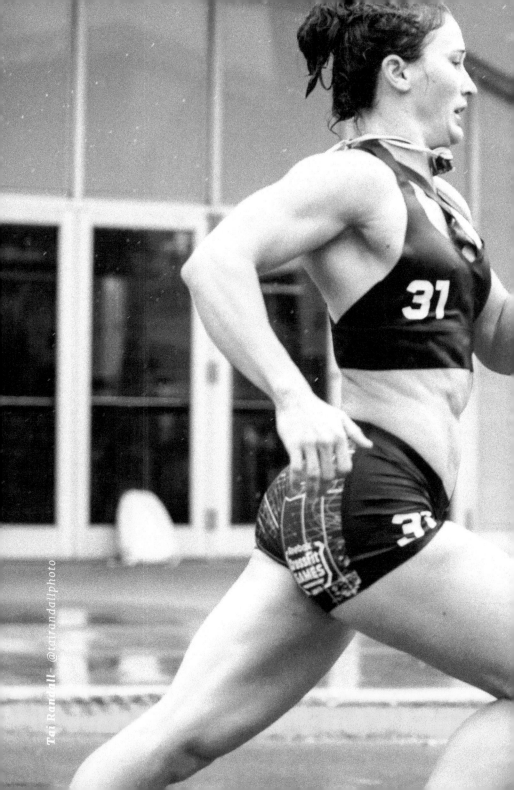

COMPETING AT THE 2017 CROSSFIT GAMES IN THE

Run. Swim. Run.

Competing at the

2017
CROSSFIT
GAMES

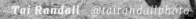

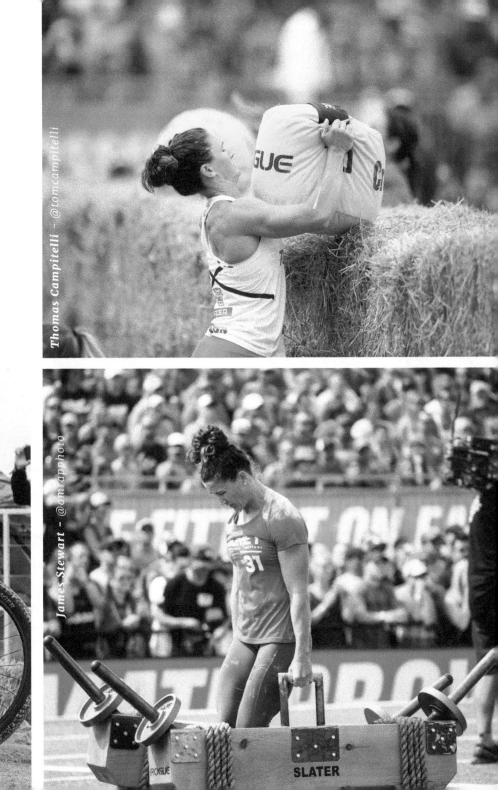

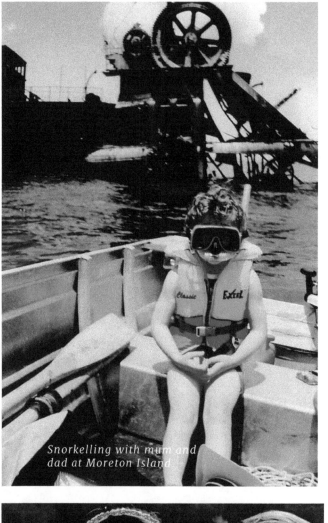

Snorkelling with mum and dad at Moreton Island

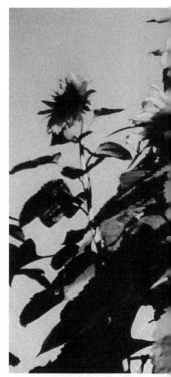

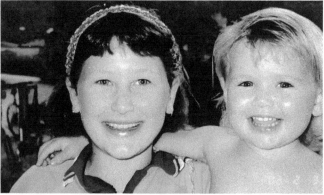

Me and my sister, Elle

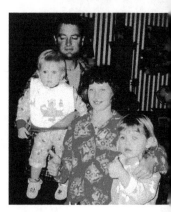

Me, my sisters and Dad

SUNFLOWERS

I planted and
grew a garden bed
of Sunflowers

(my favourite flower growing up)

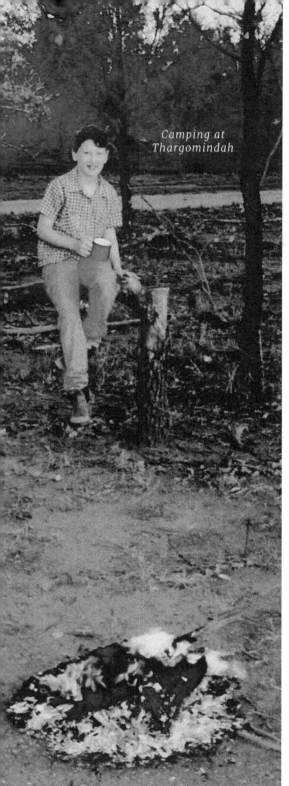

Camping at Thargomindah

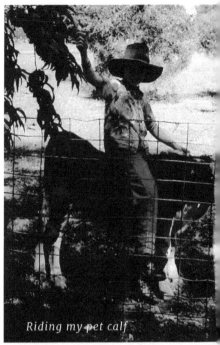

Riding my pet calf

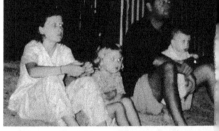

My dad, sisters and I sitting on the ramp watching the cane fires on the farm

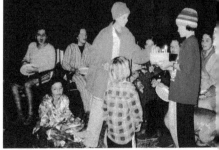

My friends and I camping on the farm for my 9th birthday

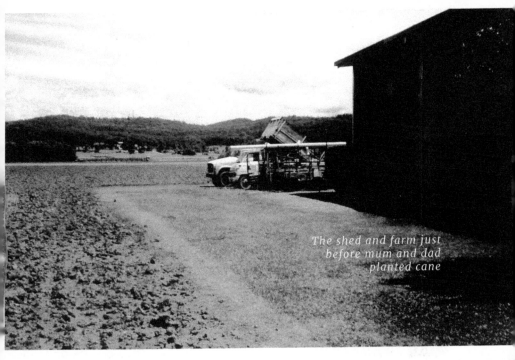

The shed and farm just before mum and dad planted cane

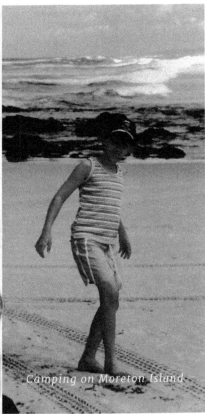

Camping on Moreton Island

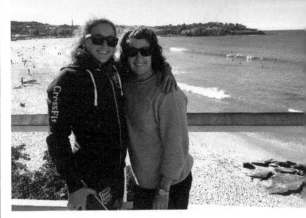

Me and mum

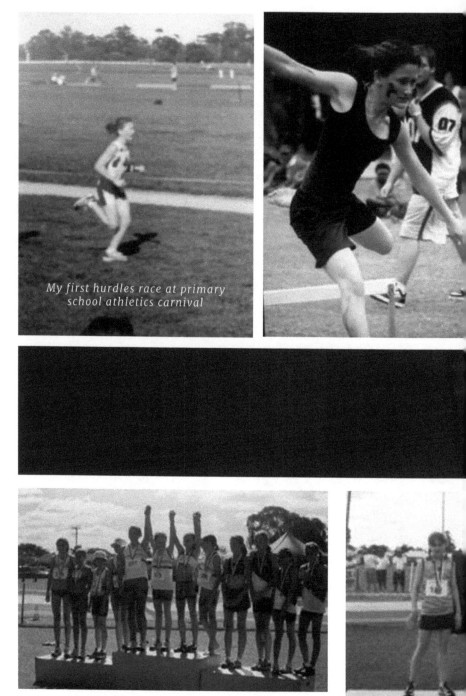

My first hurdles race at primary
school athletics carnival

My Sunshine Coast cross country team
winning our relay race at States

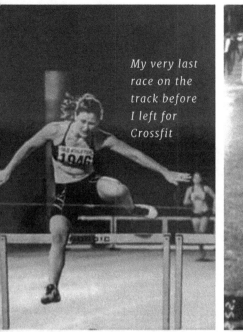

My very last race on the track before I left for Crossfit

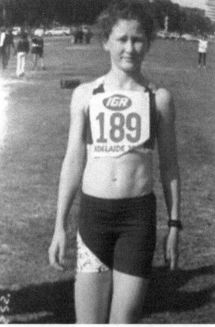

PRIMARY SCHOOL

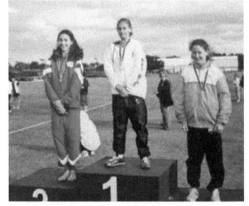

Me coming third in Maryborough for Cross Country, my first time making States

Me coming third in my cross country race at States in Townsville

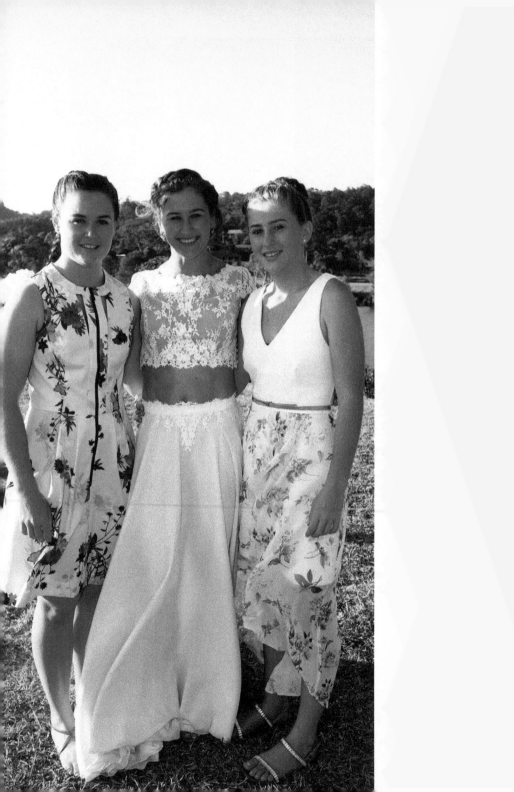

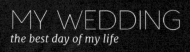

MY WEDDING
the best day of my life

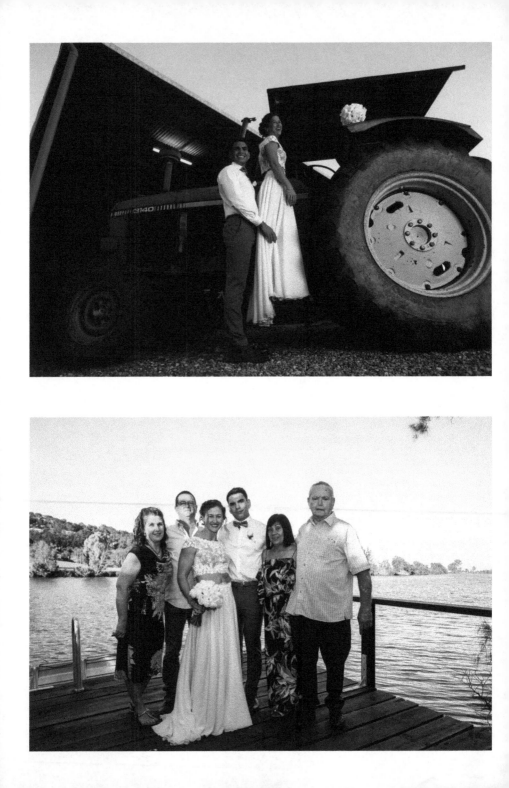

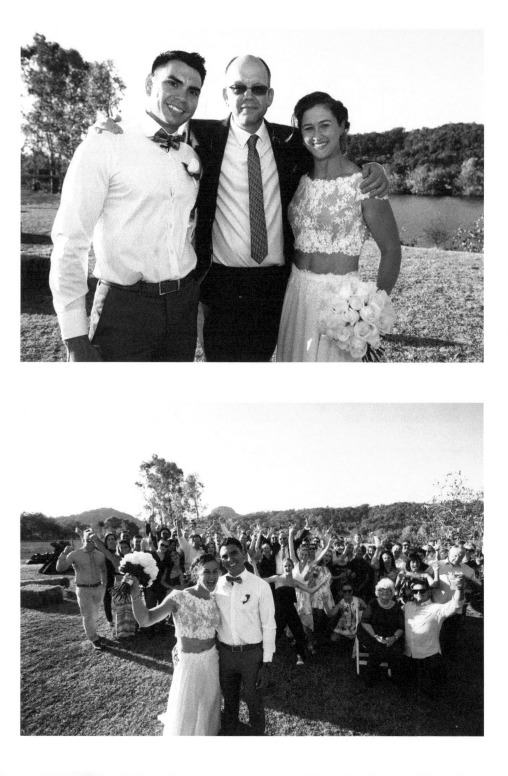

TRAINING

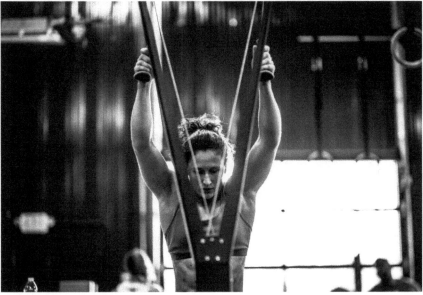

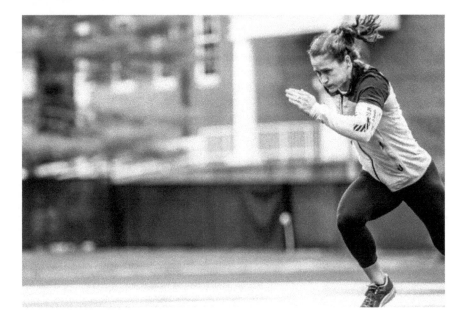

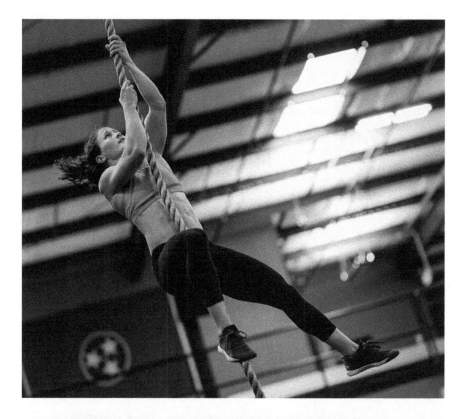

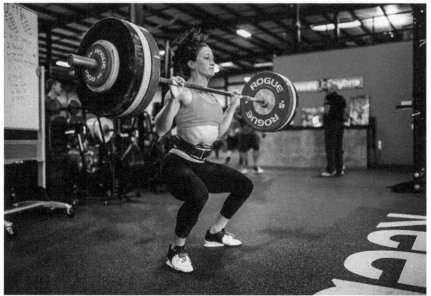

*Rio and I when we first got him once I got
announced I made the Olympics*

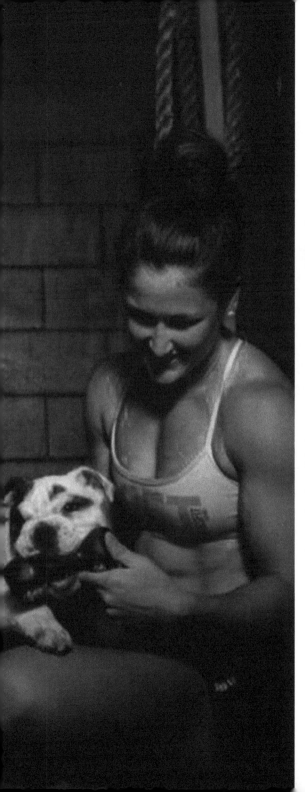

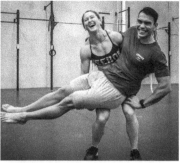

Shane and I just mucking around

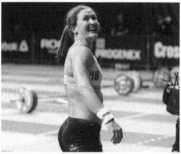

Me looking up to Shane, mum and my friends in the crowd at Regionals

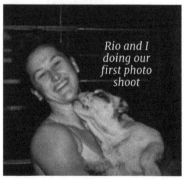

Rio and I doing our first photo shoot

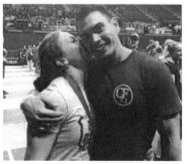

Shane and I at Regionals when I first ever made the CrossFit Games

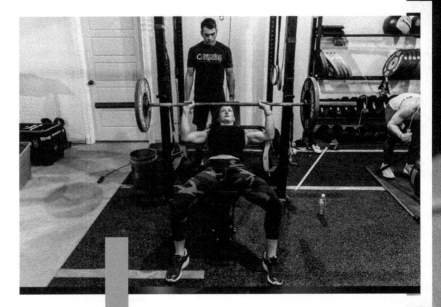

SHANE AND I
TRAINING

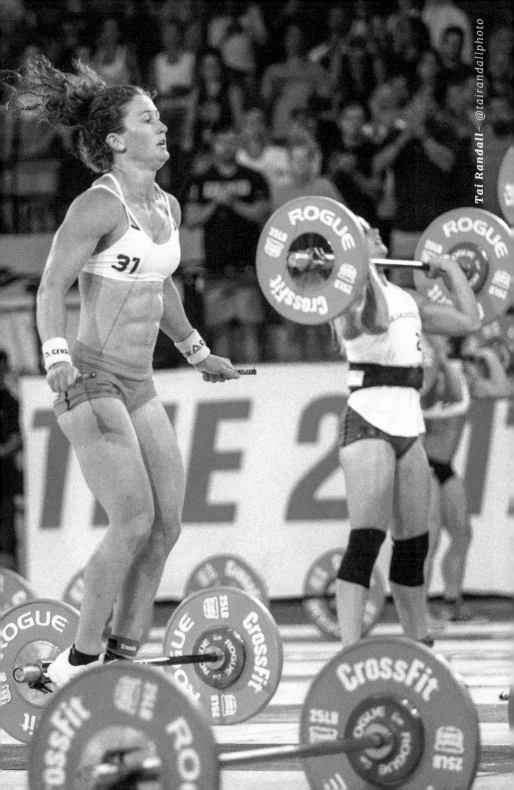

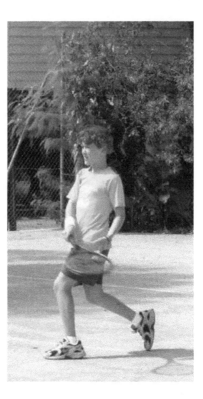

*My first
tennis
competition*

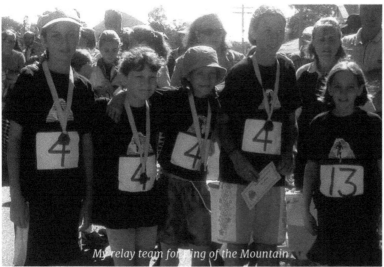

My relay team for King of the Mountain

MY
FIRST
DAY
of grade 1

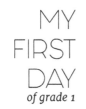

*The farm just before mum
and dad planted the sugar
cane and the river*

COMING FIRST

at my year 7 cross country

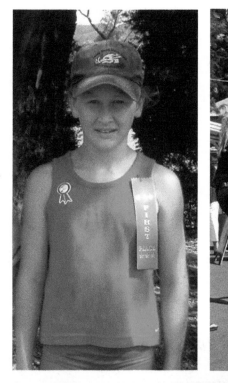

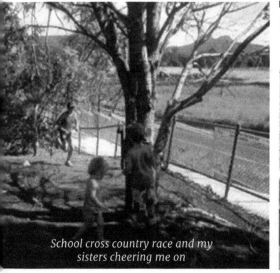

School cross country race and my sisters cheering me on

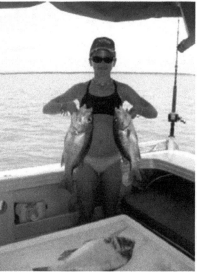

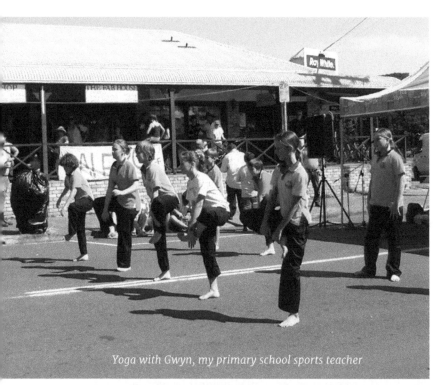

Yoga with Gwyn, my primary school sports teacher

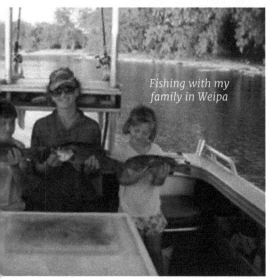

Fishing with my family in Weipa

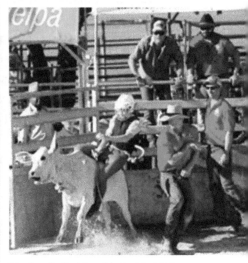

My first bull ride with Dad in Weipa

CHAPTER 15

Time to Lift

When Shane and I walk our dogs around the block at night, it's our time to talk and share what's really going on in our heads. In January 2016, my head was so full of endless 'what if?' scenarios that I couldn't think straight.

"Babe, I don't know what I am going to do if I don't make the Olympics this year. And then what happens if I can't back up my performance at the CrossFit Games? I'll feel like a failure."

"Tia, all you have to do is trust in the process and you will be successful. If I'm not worried, you shouldn't be worried."

Shane's ability to stay calm and composed in my moments of doubt has been a huge help to me over the years. Later that week, I competed and placed second at Regionals, securing my spot at the 2016 CrossFit Games which was a big relief. Next on my list was securing my spot at the Olympics at the last round of trials in Fiji one week later.

I still had a few days to settle myself before I flew out to Fiji with the Australian weightlifting team. Shane took the opportunity for us to spend some quality time together and arranged a beautiful evening on Sydney Harbour.

We went out on a sunset boat cruise and I was finding it hard to relax because all I wanted to do was get back in the gym and start prepping for the final trial. The evening turned out to be one of the most touching and heartwarming times of my life. Over a beautiful dinner in Watson's Bay, Sydney, Shane proposed to me. I was able to completely forget about CrossFit and weightlifting and spend time celebrating my biggest achievement in my life – my relationship with Shane. We ate chocolates, enjoyed a bottle of champagne and chatted the night away. It was a very special moment that I will never forget and hope that everyone in the world is lucky enough to experience that feeling of complete love and fulfillment.

The proposal brought me back to what's really important in life and that's Shane, my family and friends. I was getting too caught up in how I was going to perform rather than actually remembering why I was doing it.

I know that whatever Shane and I do and whatever we set our minds to, we will never fail. We're both the type of people who will always try our hardest and never give up. We may fail in the sense that we don't achieve a goal. However, that doesn't mean we're going to give up, we're just going to learn from it and try again. We have some sort of equation that just works, both personally and professionally. It comes down to trust, communication, respect and passion - all things we both value. I left Sydney feeling more relaxed than ever, ready to tackle Fiji and make the Olympics.

***

Athletes from 18 nations arrived in Suva, Fiji for the 2016 Oceania Weightlifting Championships. The atmosphere was tense because it was a make-or-break competition for a lot of athletes, me included.

In Olympic weightlifting, the two competition lifts are the snatch and the clean and jerk. The competition starts with each athlete naming the weight they will start on, with the lowest going first. In order to provide a total there needs to be at least one successful lift from each movement. Athletes get three attempts in each and the combined total of the highest two successful lifts determines the winner in each bodyweight category.

Since the CrossFit Games began, the interest in weightlifting has grown significantly, the most obvious reason being that the Games incorporate many weightlifting movements.

Women's weight categories start at 48 kilograms and go up in five-kilogram increments until the last weight category, which is 90 kilograms and over. The lighter weight categories always lift first so I was up on day two of the competition. It was nerve-wracking lifting early on in the piece because I had to watch and wait around a few more days to see how everyone performed before I knew if I had made the Olympics or not. And it's even more suspenseful when there is only one spot up for grabs!

'You've got this, Tia, you show them why you deserve to go to Rio. You go out there and show them what you're made of.'

I was standing in the warm up area, psyching myself up before I walked out on the floor. There were 10 or so girls in my weight category but I was focusing on the task at hand and didn't take much notice of what was happening around me. This was my last chance to secure my spot for the Olympics so whatever Miles told me to do, I did.

Shane had done his job in preparing me and Miles was the boss now. "Put 40 kilograms on the bar and do two lifts."

I gave the nod and followed my order. When preparing for a lift in weightlifting, there isn't much talking that goes on. I always try to get in the zone and visualise myself lifting while Miles concentrates on the numbers. I looked back up to Miles and he gave me the nod again, indicating I was up. I gave a little grunt, stood up and got ready to go out to the platform. Now it was my turn to do my job, to perform!

I gave it a red-hot crack and I was reasonably happy with what I lifted - a platform PB snatch and a decent clean and jerk. I always want more from myself but that was the best I could do on the day so I accepted it reluctantly. Then the waiting game began. I had to wait almost a week to see how all of the other athletes did and to find out whether I made the Olympics, which was dreadful. I was anxious because there were 10 other girls still to lift and all I could do was sit there and watch. I felt so sick. Every time I'd watch one of the girls lift, all I could think was, 'Did they beat me?' It was a weird situation to be in; I wanted the girls to perform at their best but I didn't want them to take the top spot away from me either.

Every lady who lifted in Fiji was a contender for the Olympics so I knew if I got the spot I really did go up against the best of the best. By the end of the last day, Miles told me that I had unofficially been selected for the Olympics. It was an inconceivable feeling, but it was bittersweet at the same time because it was heartbreaking for the other Aussies who didn't make it. There wasn't much celebrating afterwards because there were so many mixed emotions in the room. I definitely didn't take the opportunity for granted and knew I was going to grind harder than ever to make Australia proud.

Shane and Miles were so happy for me. We all felt relieved that our hard work had paid off. At the time of my competition, my Pop had taken a turn for the worst and was in hospital so all I wanted to do was call him and tell him my news. I almost think a part of him was holding on to hear whether I made the Olympics. He was so proud of me and would tell all of the nurses about my new success and what I was up to. Every opportunity I got when I was home I would go down to see Pop and take him out for lunch or to go hang out with his friends playing snooker and golf. It broke my heart to see him so frail because he was such a strong man.

I laid down in bed and dialed his number.

"Hello, my love."

His voice was so wispy and frail but it warmed me to hear him on the line.

"Pop, I made the Olympics! It's not official yet, so don't tell anyone, but I really did make it!"

"Oh Tia, I'm so happy for you, darling. What a year you have had."

"I know, Poppy, I know. I love you so much."

"I have such a special girl. You have achieved so much, my love. Shane proposed, you made the Games again and now the Olympics, you should be so proud."

He couldn't say much more but I could hear just how proud he was. About a week later, Pop passed away and it broke my heart. That man meant a lot to me, it was so sad to let him go. I carry his love with me every day and it's a big reason why I push harder to achieve my goals.

***

Shane always wanted a bulldog but we already had two dogs so every time he brought up the idea I deferred it. Just before Fiji, he begged again until one day I gave in and said, 'Fine, if I make the Olympics, you can get a bulldog!' The moment we got home, our family of four turned to five and Shane got his bulldog who we named Rio after the Olympic Games host city. I was home and ready to hone in on my training for the CrossFit Games and Olympics, which were only weeks away. I couldn't believe I was about to realise my dream of going to the Olympics and the CrossFit Games in the same year, it was surreal.

CHAPTER 16

Double Whammy

I am reminded of my goals at least 20 times a day because I write them on the back of my phone and have little notes around the house to keep me focused and motivated. I don't just read them, I say them out loud and I say them boldly. Our minds don't know the difference between real and imagined information. So I know if I say what I want to happen enough times, my mind will help me accomplish it.

The other key for me is repetition. It's like riding a bike; I do it so many times that one day I don't even think about it, I just do it. That's what I try to achieve with my goals - I say my goals so often and with so much conviction that they actually come to fruition.

In 2016, the problem was I had a lack of confidence in my own ability. Instead of having the courage to say, 'I want to win the CrossFit Games', I kept coming back to passive goals like 'My goal is to place second or better' or 'Just don't place worse than second.' Both goals came from such a place of self-doubt which was so unlike me. Looking back now it's no wonder I didn't win the 2016 CrossFit Games, with an attitude like that. I did an interview with a guy called James from BossFit before the Games and when he asked me what my goal was, my reply reeked of doubt.

"My goal is to make it into the top two of the Pacific region…I'm not putting any pressure on myself to have a particular overall placing in mind."

I wasn't able to admit that I wanted to win the Games because I was scared of not living up to everyone's expectations. I was sure of my physical ability but I was unsure of whether I could deliver on game day and I kept doubting myself. After the comments regarding my performance at the 2015 Games, I really started to think that those people were right, maybe my performance was a fluke. Maybe I did only come second because there were lots of running events which played to my strengths. If I was stronger mentally I would have brushed it off, but I let it get to me.

In the weeks leading up to the Games, I kept saying to Shane, 'Is this good enough? Have we done enough? Do I even have what it takes to win?' The reality is that when training for the CrossFit Games, the unpredictability is so high. The events aren't known until just hours before and there is always going to be something that really challenges. It comes down to whether athletes have the confidence in their own ability to accept the challenge and move forward.

Going into the 2016 Games, the competition was fierce and a part of me still felt like I wasn't as legit as the other athletes. I was excited for the Ranch Trail Run, having the honour of going back to where the Games began, and running in the footsteps of athletes before me. The run was particularly challenging because it was a dusty, hilly, cross-country track in the Californian sun along with 79 other runners but

I loved the challenge. I placed sixth amongst the ladies and was just glad I didn't flop in my first event. I was heading in the right direction to back up my performance.

My Mum, Dad and Shane - actually, everyone that has supported me along the way - kept saying that I could win the Games if I believed in myself, but I just didn't know if I did. When the CrossFit media would ask me questions in interviews, I kept playing myself down because I didn't want to over-promise and under-deliver, I didn't think twice about how I came across. I was stoked when the Ocean Swim was announced because I knew I could shine in it.

"I feel like I've got this one easy, Shane, this workout was made for me – it's like Nippers all over again. I'm actually excited for it!"

"Yes, Tia, this is what I've been waiting to see! You're finally backing yourself!"

It was a close finish but I took out first place and felt like I was getting to where I needed to be. Everyone was right, if I backed myself there was no stopping me. I placed first in the suicide sprints which felt almost effortless. I was feeling good all round, I had finally won a couple of events at the CrossFit Games. I stayed towards the top of the field for most of my events and my self-doubt started to dwindle away but I left my run too late.

***

The 2016 presentations were so painful. It took a ridiculously long time to determine the winner, everyone in the stadium was looking down at us on the floor. I didn't know how the placings or points would stack up and it was the most dragged-out five minutes of my life.

The moment I found out I came second, I was gutted. I thought I might have been in with a chance so the surprise stabbed me in the heart. To taste it and be so close to winning and not being able to follow through was heartbreaking. I was happy to be on the podium again but I wasn't happy with my performance. I was disappointed and thought, 'Wow, Tia, you just missed a great opportunity. You could have won it but you threw it all away because of a little self-doubt.' I wasn't at all satisfied and all I could think about was how much I had let Shane down. He lived up to his part of the deal - he coached me, programmed me, warmed me up, stretched me out, prepared my meals, heated up my meals, massaged me, wrote up my strategy. All I had to do was go out and perform and I'd stuffed it.

Deep down, I was emotionless but I couldn't let that affect my prep for the Olympics. We stopped off in Miami on our way to Rio to break the trip up. We finished training for the day in Miami and Shane suggested we go to the beach for a bit to hang out. We were swimming around in paradise and I just started crying. I didn't say anything but Shane hugged me. He knew I was still processing the loss and coming to terms with the result.

Then things got worse when I watched the 2016 CrossFit 'Fittest on Earth' documentary. I was excited to see what snippets they'd captured of me and boy, did I get a shock. It was the very first time the CrossFit media had the cameras focused on me and I remember it feeling very unnatural. I was so shy and intimidated; I didn't know how to act. I gave a lot of jovial responses to questions because I wanted to make a tense situation a bit more fun and not take myself too seriously in front of the cameras but it all came across so wrong. Everything was negative.

Watching the doco was a slap in the face. The worst part of it was when someone got a photo with me and I said, 'You might want to delete that at the end of the weekend because I won't come first!' I sounded insecure and not at all confident in my own abilities. I was really upset but it was definitely the wake-up call I needed. I lost it again to Shane, I was so ashamed.

"This is the first year I've ever been on camera and this is how I come across. All of my friends and family know I'm not like that but the whole world thinks I am. How does that even happen? I just don't understand, I am such a fool."

Shane comforted me and said all the right things to ease my mind and when I spoke to Mum, all I cared about was keeping my sisters from seeing it.

"Please don't show my sisters, Mum. I'm so mortified. If they see it, I'm showing them that it's okay to beat yourself down. I don't want them to see me weak like that."

I know the media guys didn't intend any malice and at the end of the day, those words came out of my mouth so I had no one else to blame but myself. It was definitely a learning curve for me; to never again talk myself down, even if I was just mucking around.

***

Shane and I met Miles in Rio and started prepping for competition day, which was only two weeks after competing at the CrossFit Games. My lead-up to the competition was the best it had ever been, my nutrition was dialled in to the tee, I cut my weight easily and I hit my competition weights for both the snatch and clean and jerk.

My expectations going into Rio were completely different to the CrossFit Games. I wanted to go out there and give it my all, without any attachment to a specific placing. This goal didn't come from a place of self-doubt but aiming to get a medal would have been impossible for me, given the competition I was up against. That didn't stop me from wanting to train hard and attempt to PB my lifts on the world stage.

There is no denying the Olympics is the pinnacle of all sporting events and to be an Olympian is a dream come true for me. I was able to stay in prime condition - unhurt and injury free - which was another bonus. I couldn't have been in better shape.

I felt so proud at the Australian flag-raising in the Olympic Village, to be surrounded by the sporting greats of the world and listen to their speeches was nothing short of unbelievable. When I changed into my suit ready to compete, I was honoured to wear the green and gold and be there representing my country.

Shane, Mum and Disey all came to support me and walking onto the Olympic platform in front of my family was a very proud moment. I lifted 82 kilograms in the snatch, which was a little less than what I had hoped for, and then it was time for the clean and jerk. My personal best was 111 kilograms and after successful first and second attempts, I attempted 112 kilograms but failed in my jerk. I placed fourteenth out of 16 lifters in my weight class. I felt a little bit disappointed that I didn't beat my PBs but I really did give it my absolute best.

Having the opportunity to meet so many inspiring athletes and seeing them compete in their chosen sports was very special and the closing ceremony was full of goosebump moments.

Flying back home on the plane, I felt satisfied. I had accomplished the goal I had set out to achieve; competing at the CrossFit Games and the Olympics in the same year. The bonus was that I podiumed at the CrossFit Games so that then opened up a whole new goal for me. I wanted to do even better next year.

CHAPTER 17

My Routine

My life is all about routine. Not an insanely strict routine with rule books that are 100 pages long but a sustainable routine, with a good underlying structure that is easy to follow and adapt to the ebb and flow of life. At home, I get up every morning at 4 am if I am coaching at the gym, or 7 am if Shane is coaching. I go to the toilet and weigh myself to make sure I'm not fluctuating in weight. I have my vitamins and supplements first thing, and then make my green smoothie so I know I've had my greens for the day.

I have an immune booster, two fish oils, bio magnesium, D3 and glucosamine. My breakfast changes but my favourites are bacon, eggs and avocado on two pieces of sourdough toast or granola with fruit and Greek yogurt. After breakfast, it's time for me to sweat. I will be active for two hours outside of the gym which can be anything from swimming and walking the dogs to running or even riding my bike. Sometimes my running is on an athletics track or sometimes it's on a trail, cross-country style. As long as I'm mixing it up and have variety, I'm happy.

Then it's time for lunch! My go-to meal is steak, salad and brown rice. Sometimes I mix it up with leftovers from the night before because I like to have flexibility in my eating. I know it's recommended to have more routine and have set meal plans and food diaries, but for me, being too regimented wears too thin. I know that if I ate chicken and broccoli day in and day out I would burn out and get over it. If I restrict myself from eating certain foods, it takes the joy out of my life. Obviously, I'm not going to have a Big Mac every day but a nutritious stir-fry or healthy curry isn't going to hinder my performance or recovery. This approach just aligns to my career philosophy of enjoying the journey.

After lunch, I usually get on my computer and attend to emails and work for CrossFit Gladstone. If I want to have time out from work, I watch TV while I stretch and try and prep the body for my afternoon session in the gym. I make sure I have a protein bar or a piece of fruit and a coffee before I head to the gym, just to give me an extra bit of energy and something to look forward to before training.

My afternoon session is three, sometimes four, hours long and we start at about two o'clock in the afternoon. I take my protein shake, towel and water bottle and head to CrossFit Gladstone. I like to ease into my sessions and start with a slow stretch. There is always a bit of banter between Shane, myself and some of our mates that train with us, Travy and Will. We write up our routine on the whiteboard and get started. Our workouts vary but they will always have some sort of strength and technical barbell component, skill and gymnastics component and a couple of metcon and conditioning components. Towards the end of my training session, Shane usually has to leave early and start coaching the evening CrossFit classes and Travy, Will and I will finish off with my accessories.

After coaching, Shane and I head home at about 8.45 pm, walk the dogs around and sit down to have dinner. I have almost put Shane in hospital with food poisoning from my cooking and have been banned from the kitchen, so he generally cooks dinner unless we go out for a social dinner with friends. No matter where I am, as long as I have a good source of protein, carbohydrate and fats in my meals then I'm happy. I follow that same principle for all of my meals to make sure I'm hitting my macros. It also allows me to ensure I am consuming quality food and not over-eating.

It doesn't matter how late it is, I always sit down on the couch at the end of each day for at least half an hour to switch off and enjoy just chilling out. I go to bed pretty late, usually around 10.30 pm but I try to get a minimum of seven hours sleep. Sometimes this is hard to achieve when I have to coach at 4 am but I do my best because I know I function so much better on seven to eight hours a night. The main reason I have late nights is because I train so much, so I need to have time in between to recover properly. There is no point in me doing all of that volume if I'm not doing it properly, it's not effective and that's when injuries happen. So, in order to train properly, I have longer days.

***

Early on in my career, I always thought that if I treated myself with chocolate or sweets, it would result in me not being successful in achieving my goals which is not the case. Once I realised that I could treat myself after a long day and still stay within my macros and maximise my recovery for the next day of training, I began to implement treats. It made me feel so much more content and gave me drive to work harder. Sometimes I'd say to myself, 'If you don't push hard you don't deserve it but if you go like hell and walk out of the gym with no regrets, then you can have your treat.' It doesn't affect my performance and it gives me the satisfaction that I'm actually living a normal life like everyone else. That is the most important key to having a long, enjoyable career.

I keep my food intake pretty similar during competition, the only real difference is I eat a lot of pureed food straight after a workout, so the nutrients hit my body faster to help with recovery. If I have a long three-hour period in between an event, I will immediately eat a meal straight after so my body can prepare itself. I also am very conscious of eating too much protein during competition because my body uses a lot of energy to break protein down so I'm always looking for carbs and fats.

Depending on the time of year, my training volume changes from one session a day to three sessions a day and Shane's the one that makes the call. It's such an advantage having him as my coach because he can read my body language and energy levels in the gym and at home. Sometimes I don't even need to say anything. He just knows, which is the beauty of living together and being a team. He knows how much sleep I'm getting and what food I'm eating so if something isn't working, he knows what to adjust without having to ask.

CHAPTER 18

On a Mission

That empty feeling of failure after a loss stuck with me all the way until the 2017 CrossFit Games. I felt so disappointed that I didn't fight harder for first place the year before. All I wanted was to be number one and going into 2017, I wasn't afraid to tell anyone and everyone, 'I want to win the CrossFit Games.'

At the start of each year, Shane and I make adjustments to our lifestyle to free up more time to prioritise training for the Games and weightlifting. When I was away competing in 2015 and 2016, I would continually check in with CrossFit Gladstone to make sure all of the back-end work was being completed. I still had a business to run and I didn't want my members feeling abandoned while I was overseas. I was doing membership requests, updating my books and making sure everything was still running smoothly. I was operating in so many different worlds that my mind wasn't focused solely on competing.

In January 2017, we started to change things around. We redirected a lot of our priorities and cut back on things to make training for the 2017 Games our priority. We didn't cut back on everything - so that we became too consumed by the Games - but enough to ensure I was more focused. I don't view changes as sacrifices, I see them as adjustments that need to happen in order to achieve a bigger picture.

Shane quit his job at the gas plant and took over my managing role at CrossFit Gladstone so I could dedicate more time to my own training. We bought a sauna that we put in our living room to help with my recovery, I started getting regular massages from a professional masseuse and I prepared all of my food the day before so I could eat straight after my training. It wasn't that these things helped me win but they certainly helped me get in the zone.

One thing that we didn't adjust was how and when we trained at our gym. Our members' classes were still our number one priority and we continued to change my training schedule to suit our clients.

Shane reached out to coaches from various sports to see what he could learn from them and apply to my training, particularly with regards to technique. Shane is very good at taking suggestions and learning from other coaches in different fields. It means he's always evolving as a coach and keeping his finger on the pulse in every way possible. But when it comes down to crunch time at the Games and taking on words of advice, Shane is the only person I want in my corner. When we set out on the CrossFit Games journey, we wanted to achieve the ultimate goal of us on top of the podium together. We were determined the journey would be about us as a partnership and wanted to see how far we could go without any other coaches involved.

***

We were only three months out from the Games and I was going through a low period, constantly bringing myself down. I held such a high standard for myself because I knew from experience what it took to win.

"I'm not happy with today, Shane. I just don't feel like I'm getting any better."

"Was that the best you could do?"

"No, I could have done better yesterday if I trained in the morning when I was fresh."

"Forget yesterday, Tia, it's today! Just trust the process, we are doing everything we need to do to get to where we want to be."

"I expect better, I expect more from myself. Getting a PB isn't good enough, Shane. I know I can get more, I want more for me!"

"All I ask from you as a coach right now is the best you can give me in this moment under the current circumstances, that's it."

No matter what Shane said or what I did, I was stuck in a rut of doubt. I kept saying to myself after every training session, 'Is that really the best you can do, Tia?' I was messing with my own head, playing weird mind games with myself.

As the CrossFit Games got closer my emotions started going up and down like rollercoaster, I didn't know if I was Arthur or Martha. There were times when I was frustrated to tears with myself and my training performances. And then there were other times when I thought, 'I'm killing it.' I was all over the place.

***

In most sports, athletes get to compete against their competition throughout the season. It's different when it comes to the CrossFit Games - there is only one opportunity to scout out the competition and that's at the Games itself. Not only are the abilities of the competitor's relatively unknown, but the style and number of events differs every year and the workouts are only announced two hours before they commence. With so many unknowns, it's only natural to feel some sort of uncertainty or doubt and ask yourself, 'How do you even train for this?' After training, I often think, 'I hope Shane knows what he's doing. I trust him to no end but is he overlooking something? Is he covering everything?' As hard as it is not knowing what events lay ahead, the mystery of the Games is also what makes it so fun and challenging!

Shane and I did do some pretty out-of-the-box things in preparation for the 2017 CrossFit Games. One day, Shane made a spur-of-the-moment decision to book us into a rowing session on the Fitzroy River in Rockhampton. We drove an hour and a half to the river and did a two-hour rowing session. I'd never done it before and wasn't too sure about it.

"Shane, the Games are two months away and we're wasting a whole day driving in the car to go rowing on the off-chance that there's rowing at the Games. I just think this is a waste of time, if I'm honest."

"It's not just about the Games, T, it will be nice for us to mix it up and go against the grain a little!"

The setting was beautiful and weather was perfect. We rowed down the picturesque river and I felt my stresses float away. As usual, Shane was on the money. The rowing was a great experience and I couldn't believe how much I learnt about balance. I needed more control and balance on the water compared to a rowing machine and had to focus on activating my core so much more. Regardless of whether there was rowing at the Games or not, the exercise was relaxing, centering and taught me important new skills. It was worthwhile after all.

There were also rumours circulating before the 2017 Games that a biathlon was going to be incorporated into one of the events. Biathlon combines cross-country skiing and rifle shooting. I think us Australians would have been the most disadvantaged in that event, given skiing isn't exactly one of our most popular past-times. With this in mind, Shane and I decided to go to a rifle range on our way to the Games so we could practice our aim in a shooting range. We didn't seriously think it would be an event but you never know and we thought after the rowing experience, 'Why not do it for fun?!'

There really are no limits or guidelines with the Games. If it can be classified as a sport on some level then you can bet your bottom dollar in some way, shape or form, one day it will make its way into the Games. There is always one unusual event at the CrossFit Games that the majority of athletes would have never even heard of before. I absolutely love the surprise of it and count down for them to announce it each year. As part of the unusual event, Rogue, the equipment sponsor of the Games, brings out a new piece of equipment that no one has seen or touched before. The equipment and the movements are never normal and athletes have to adjust on the fly and drive themselves through the race the best way they can. I love how the Games challenges me to compete against other athletes at the same time as it challenges me in my own life – I get pushed on a personal level to go way out of my comfort zone and attack things I never thought were possible.

Really, it doesn't matter how many things you hypothesise that the Games organisers may or may not do, fitness will prevail. Shane could get me to do crazy things in the lead-up to the Games, like a sauna workout or putting on a ridiculously heavy vest and running five miles in the heat but I would rather not cook my body and totally dehydrate myself. I would rather just keep my training to the fundamentals; run, swim, bike to get fit and lift, pull, push to get strong and like to think I will do alright.

***

We headed over to the US just over two weeks before the 2017 Games began. I organised to train with another CrossFit athlete, one of the male competitors, Josh Bridges. He's a four-time Games veteran and a former US Navy Seal, so comes from a background of mental toughness and his pain threshold is through the roof! Training with

Josh is a great way for me to throw my usual programming out the window and do something completely different. It makes me train in a different environment with different people where I don't have control over anything. I thrive off Josh's intensity and training with him really does provide me with the best preparation possible.

At our last training session, Josh was pumping me up and helping me build my self-confidence even more.

"Tia, when you're in the middle of a workout and you're feeling that pain more than ever and all you want to do is give in, just ask yourself 'If they can do it, then why can't I?' If you're hurting, then the chances are your competitors are hurting more than you."

Josh is the master of pushing through pain and I will never forget what he told me about his time as a Navy Seal.

"When my Commander used to ask us questions, his response was 'GOOD!' He saw pain as a good thing. He'd say:
'How is the pain?'
'It hurts Sir.'
'GOOD!'
'Is it hard?'
'Yes, Sir.'
'GOOD!'"

He was right. The pain is a positive feeling and I had to embrace it. Josh said one other thing to me while I was stretching down on our last day of training.

"Tia, lesser people have won the CrossFit Games, so why can't you?"

All of Josh's words resonated with me, those ones especially. That saying stayed in my head throughout every single workout in the 2017 CrossFit Games.

After five days in San Diego training with Josh, Shane and I flew to Chicago then drove to Madison, Wisconsin, to get our routine in gear one week out from the Games. For the first time, we didn't have to think or worry about the gym back home. All eyes were on the prize. It was like we were on vacation but a vacation to train and win.

CHAPTER 19

Games Warm-Up

After competing in California the previous years, I was pumped to see all of the new courses and facilities in Madison. The events were set up in different areas spread out across more than 160 acres of land and the quality of equipment was unbelievable.

On the Monday morning, we hired bikes and embarked on an active recovery ride before heading to the stadium for registration. We collected Shane's coaching pass and my athlete credential pass and walked through to the Reebok area to get kitted up. Reebok gave all the athletes a big bag with an endless supply of clothes and shoes, branded with everyone's name and number. This is always one of the exciting parts of the CrossFit Games, I love getting so many different items of shoes and apparel. We were totally spoilt. Reebok even had seamstresses sitting in stations ready to make alterations to people's gear that didn't fit properly. The attention to detail was amazing.

Shane and I continued down the big hallway and got to the shoes station. Once my foot was measured properly, Andreas from Reebok handed over eight pairs of shoes for every occasion; there were workout shoes, stylish streetwear shoes, lifting shoes, runners, speeds and a one-off shoe designed especially for the unusual event. We balanced all my bags on either side of our bodies and continued walking towards a sea of sponsors eagerly waiting to hand over more free stuff. I got given a 15-kilogram dumbbell, supplements, shakers, sunglasses and protein powder, the gifts just kept coming. Because I am a Reebok athlete, we received hand-painted Reebok Classics as a gift for making the Games. They really did go all out for us. By the end of registration, we all walked away looking like we had just cleaned up at a massive Boxing Day sale.

I took everything back to the room and got ready for the Spectacle Dinner with Dave Castro. The dinner is the first proper opportunity to meet and catch up with all the other athletes. It's tradition for Dave to announce some movements or one of the workouts at the dinner so athletes get a sneak peek before the Games begin. We all met at the hotel and walked over to the restaurant. Everyone was so excited to catch up and talk all things CrossFit Games. Sara Sigmundsdottir, Sam Briggs and I found a seat and settled in ready for Dave's big announcement. He stood up with a huge grin on his face, waiting in silence for everyone's attention.

"I want to congratulate everyone for making it this far. This is going to be an exciting year because we are in a different venue that opens up a world of new opportunities. I'm very excited about what we have in store for you this year. It is going to be the hardest and most challenging year to date, so I hope you're ready."

Dave is amazing at commanding the attention of a room. We were all fixated on him and what he was about to reveal. There were laughs and giggles from all the veterans who had heard the same speech from Dave a number of times before while all of the rookies were sitting in fear thinking, 'What have I got myself into?'

"If you haven't come here to win, then I suggest you walk out of those doors now because I am here to find the Fittest Man and Woman on Earth. I can tell you that one of the events we have created especially for this year's Games is ... actually, I'm not going to tell you, let's show you!"

Dave sat back down and the room started buzzing. Everyone was talking about the new information and speculating about what the event could be. The TVs in the restaurant turned on and we were all glued to the screens. Some athletes had their phones out recording it and some athletes were writing notes.

The film featured a professional athlete demonstrating the course. It was on a grass track and had a lot of sharp turns. We didn't really know what sport we were watching but knew it was bike-riding of some sort. Halfway through the video, the experienced bike rider jumped off his bike and carried it over some small hurdles and across a pit of sand then got back on the bike and continued to ride.

Once the film was over, Dave announced that we were going to be doing a Cyclocross event on day one and on Wednesday - the day before event one - we all had to do a time trial to determine where we would start the race. You could hear the rumour mill gaining more momentum. No one knew how they would perform in such a left-of-centre event.

Shane tells me that social media during the Games gets out of control with rumours and banter circulating across the world. During the Games, I stay away from social media to maintain focus. Every now and then Shane monitors it for me and reads out the messages of support I receive from family and friends and helps me reply to my supporters. My fans and supporters mean everything to me, the fact that they take time out of their busy lives to send their well wishes to me is incredible. I am so thankful to them for backing me and my journey.

***

First thing the next morning, Shane and I went to the local bike shop to hire two bikes to practice for the Cyclocross event. Even though we knew the bike would be different to the bike in the Games, it didn't matter. We wanted to practice the fundamentals of getting on and off the bike and transitioning smoothly. We went down to a local park and practiced all morning. We found some logs to mirror the hurdles we had to jump over while carrying the bike. There was a lot of trial and error but Shane helped me navigate the important parts.

"As long as you get off the bike in the same gear you want to be in when you get back on the bike, then you will be fine."

I trialled lots of different gears but third gear gave me the perfect amount of leverage to explode.

"Just keep in mind when you get off and on the bike, you want everything to be as fluid as possible. You want to be in motion going forwards the entire time, don't stop when you transition."

I was so glad we did the trial because there was no way I would have been able to do the race blind. I would have spent the first half finding my feet. As we did laps around the park we passed a lot of the other athletes doing the same thing, each strategising and practicing in their own way.

I was pretty buggered from our day of training but we had to get ready for the coaches and athletes sponsor dinner that night. It was a Mexican buffet with all the good stuff and provided an opportunity for the sponsors to promote themselves. The most exciting part of the night for an athlete is when Dave gets up on stage and uncovers all of the Rogue equipment for the next few days. The equipment is laid out on the stage with big tarps on top to create the suspense of unveiling it. Everyone is allowed to look at the equipment and get close to it but no one is allowed to touch it. Dave called everyone in closer to gather around.

"Right, so in one of the workouts the athletes will use these large synthetic hay bales that they will jump over." I was so excited and leant over to whisper in Shane's ear.

"Hell yeah, bringing back the farm days."

Shane smiled and squeezed my hand and Dave continued on with his spiel.

"Because the Games are held here in Madison, we wanted to incorporate a bit of history, hence the hay bales. This fantastic place is also known for their cheese, so we have made a cheese curd for you to throw over the hay bales. You will run 450 metres, then perform seven hay bale clean burpees with this yellow 70-pound cheese curd sandbag."

It was an unusual concept, but fun and exciting nonetheless. He announced a few more events, some individual and some team. As every event was announced, it instilled more and more confidence in me that Shane and I had tapped into the right things throughout the season.

***

The next day was the Cyclocross time trial so we made sure we got an early night. The trial was similar to Formula One, where each competitor's lap trial determines where they start. I wasn't a strong bike rider and I didn't know how well the 40 other women rode bikes but I turned out to be not so bad. I placed sixth in the lap trial overall.

It was also a relief because there were so many potential mishaps that could happen in an event like that; someone could fall off their bike or trip over the hurdles or run into each other. And it only takes cocking up one event to ruin everything. Lots of times I've been in a race where girls in front of me have stuffed up and made a simple mistake which has enabled me to take over and cost them the event. One major slip-up and you can find yourself chasing the pack for the rest of the competition. The Fittest on Earth at the end of the day should be the most consistent athlete. That's why in 2017, two of my goals were to not place any lower than tenth and to finish all of my workouts.

CHAPTER 20

Crossfit Games

On the first day of the Games, I woke up feeling ready to make my mark but also nervous that the big day had finally arrived. I was looking forward to the first event, the Run Swim Run, because it involved my two favourite things. A lot of the other girls were strong runners as well, so I needed a decent strategy behind me.

"Remember, Tia, the race isn't won in the first run but you still need a good start so you're not playing catch up."

I kept at the front of the pack for the duration of the race and tried to stay close to the guys, who were racing at the same time as us. Coming out of the water, I could feel Kristi Eramo right next to me. I pipped her on the finish line the last year so I knew she would be expecting a late sprint from me again. I was pushing so hard and knew my splits would have be some of the fastest running I had ever done but I wasn't letting the pace affect me. I wanted those 100 points badly and I had them in my sights. I tried to put a surge in early but she hung in there. I tried again and then again, but I couldn't shake her. I remember thinking to myself, 'Make sure you save some for the end because Kristi is going to bring it'. I could hear her breathing hard and I knew she was hurting just as much as I was which gave me the drive to keep pushing through. I could see the finish line approaching and made my move before it was too late. I kicked into 'fight or flight' mode and fought hard to get over that finish line in first place, just behind the men's winner, Brent Fikowski.

The first event was done and I was ready for the next challenge. My focus was on food so that my body could recover and have enough energy to get me through to the end of the day. I had a pureed sweet potato sachet straight after the event to keep me going.

An hour later, we were on the Cyclocross track. I was a bit frustrated when I found out I was racing in the first heat. It was a massive disadvantage because the other girls in heat two could watch and learn from our mistakes and had a time to beat. The first lap was wobbly but I got in the groove by the second. There was a massive gap between me and first place but I didn't care. I just stayed composed and tried not to lose my position. All of a sudden, Bethany Brando, who had been tracking in front of me, ran into a wall and fell off her bike. I couldn't believe it. She got back on but I started making progress on her. 'Go, Tia, go, you've got to pump those legs, Tia, go, go, go!' I was pumping myself up.

We approached the sand and I jumped off my bike and pushed it along the ground instead of carrying it. I saw that Jamie Green did that on her first lap and it was way more efficient. Bethany continued to carry hers and I took over. I kept pedalling to the end and made it across the line ahead of Bethany, placing eighth overall. I was happy with my performance and the way I made up for lost time.

After the first two workouts, Dave announced we would be heading into the Coliseum for the third workout of the day, 'Amanda'. Walking into the main stadium I got goose bumps. The set-up was phenomenal and the crowd was alive, it all started to sink in and feel real. Regionals had a similar workout to 'Amanda' where I made some silly mistakes so I was ready to redeem myself. I was far too aggressive last time around so my plan was to pace myself and play my own game. I kept saying to myself, 'Be smart in your own movements, Tia, don't try and stay with the others, it's only early on. Trust your strategy, just stick to the game plan.'

I repeated this to myself over and over for the first three rounds, then I started to notice I was gaining on everyone else. There were a few of us losing the other girls and separating ourselves. I felt really composed and in the zone. Jamie Green's singles started getting faster than Samantha Briggs' and I overtook Sam and moved into second place. I was breathing down Jamie's neck but she kept strong. I paused again just before my last round which was critical in keeping my second-place position. I finished strong and Shane was so happy to see me execute the things we spoke about. We got back to our room. I crashed out straight after Shane cooked us dinner and slept like a log.

Sprint-O-Course was the first workout of the second day and I was excited but apprehensive at the same time because there was little room for error. It was very windy and a bit rainy so navigating the course was even harder. I made it through the heats to the semis but only just. It was slippery on the equipment and I lost my footing on one of the logs which cost me getting into the finals. I was too overcautious. If I wanted to make it through, I had to be aggressive but I was so hesitant. All I could think about was rolling my ankle or landing funny and ending up injured. I don't usually let those thoughts creep into my mind when I'm competing but I had too many stomach-drop moments where I felt like my ankle went that I had to play it safe. The last thing I wanted to do was hurt myself and have to pull out altogether.

I was happy to be back in the Coliseum for the rest of the day and I was so ready to snatch. I looked for Shane in the crowd and spotted his yellow kangaroo flag. I used his guidance from afar for my weight increments just to make sure I didn't make any bad calls. I made it through to the finals and went out the back quickly to speak to Shane about my next two lifts.

"Babe, my lifts felt so strong, I think I'm going to go for 95kg/209lb."
"Hang on, Tia, you have two lifts. We need to play the game and make sure you place as good as you can. Let's be a little more conservative and think about placing well rather than over-committing and not placing at all. I want you to hit 92kg/202lb, and then if you get that you can go for whatever you want."

I was confident that 92kg/202lb would be a strong lift and would put me high up on the leaderboard. Even if I didn't win, Shane had a point, I'd still be right up there and those top points are crucial.

My PB was 90kg which had I lifted in training so I had never snatched 92kg/202lb before. The crowd was roaring and firing me up big time. 'Okay, stay focused, Tia, you've got this.' I took three deep breaths, went out there and ripped that bar off the floor like nobody's business. 'YES!' I was so happy. Kara successfully lifted 203lb straight after me. I attempted 205lb but I just didn't punch that bar into the sky enough. I failed it in front, meaning I placed second to Kara.

"Awesome, T, you just need to keep building from here and keep placing consistently."

"Yep, I know, consistency is everything."

***

I had rolled my ankle badly coming down a rope climb in training a few weeks before the CrossFit Games, so my mobility was pretty bad and it showed in Triple-G Chipper, especially in my pistols. I did the workout in training and killed it but because of my poor technique I kept getting 'no rep' from the judge. I lost my composure and stuffed up the entire workout. There was absolutely nothing positive to be said between Shane and me after the event.

"What was that? You did one whole minute faster in training?!"

"I know, I just cracked under pressure, and the more I tried the more I got 'no rep'."

"You came twelfth; you really can't afford to do that again, Tia."

I knew I couldn't. My goal was to place no less then tenth place in any event and I already placed twelfth twice. Little did I know it was going to get worse before it got better.

I like the assault bike however, when I compare myself to the other girls, I'm a lot slower so knowing it was a big part of the next workout, the Assault Banger event was pretty daunting. My lungs were burning and my legs felt like jelly, I was pushing to my absolute limits but it still wasn't good enough. I actually remember thinking, 'Go Tia, you're crushing it, you might actually have a chance here', but the other girls were already off and I still had four calories to go on the bike. I just couldn't match up to the other girls. I placed fourteenth which wasn't favourable but I knew I couldn't have done better so I was happy enough.

On day three, Shane and I projected there were about six events left to go with a potential 600 points still up for grabs. I placed seventh is the next event, Strongman's Fear, which I was stoked with. After that event, I wasn't afraid of anything. I blitzed the Muscle-Up Clean Ladder, coming first by a large margin. In training, I always focus on strengthening my core because I don't like wearing a belt if I don't have to. I try not to rely on any additional equipment when I'm training as I would hate to rely on something like a belt and then, for some unknown reason, not have access to it during competition.

The Heavy 17.5 event was a repeat workout from the Open. I was so excited because I don't normally prioritise the Open at the beginning of the year because I have other commitments happening at the same time and that has been my members' time to shine. For myself, I tend to place little importance on the Open leaderboard so this was a perfect opportunity to showcase to everyone what I'm actually capable of in an Open workout.

Heavy 17.5 is an event everyone could do with their eyes closed but it came down to who wanted it more. I got off to a good start and pushed through the thrusters and double-unders. The more rounds we got through, the more Kara and I broke away from the rest of the girls. It was like it was us against the rest. Kara had a seven-second lead as we approached the finish but her arms were giving in, I almost had her. I felt so strong but fell short. Kara took her third win of the Games and I came behind in a close second place.

Kara and I hugged and she leaned into me.

"You made me push really hard then, Tia, well done."

That workout was a very proud moment for us as Australians because we pushed each other so hard, probably the hardest we have ever pushed, and it felt like it was us against the world.

Shane helped get me in the right frame of mind over breakfast. We broke everything down and he went over the plan of attack with me. "Today is the day, T; if you solidify great results on the final day and are consistent then I am confident you've got it. Just make sure above all else, you focus on your game and no one else's."

The Madison Triplet was the first workout on Sunday and I knew I could beat the people I needed to beat in order to separate myself on the leaderboard. I just had to place as high as I could to accumulate as many points possible. It was ideal that I could get the ball rolling on the final day with another running event. I was excited because it was the event with the hay bales, which made me get a bit nostalgic about the farm I grew up on.

'Holy crap, this is harder than I thought.' The burpees really got the heart rate up which made the run even harder but there was no stopping now. I got to the fourth round and made eye contact with Sam, one of our best mates who was watching on in the crowd. He was cheering for me as loud as he could.

"You've got to move! You've got to move, Tia!"

All I could think was 'I'm trying! I'm trying as hard as I can to get through this.' I crossed the finish line in third place, so short of breath it hurt. I had straw all over me, in my eyes, my mouth, even down my pants, it was everywhere. To go with it, I had a bruised, swollen shin on the right side from constantly jumping over the bales. The physical exertion was starting to take its toll.

After the Madison Triplet, I had to clean myself up and have a shower to remove all the straw before moving back into the Coliseum for the rest of the day's workouts. Shane and I didn't know how many more events we had to go but we guessed there would be around two or three as Dave always loves to put a spin on things. All of the athletes were told to head down to the basement of the Coliseum where there was warm-up gear for us to use instead of heading back to our main area.

Once 2223 Intervals was announced, nerves started to rise once again but I couldn't let any intimidation or doubt creep in. I was so close and I wasn't going to let another repeat of last year happen. I like rope climbs and overhead squats and 7 calories on the ski was nothing so I was confident I could hold my own against the other girls. I did think to myself 'Overhead Squats are Kara's jam so I need to make sure I get out in front and try to hold her off.' I went out on a pace I thought was fast enough but realised halfway through that I was already behind the mark that Shane and I had planned. From there, I was playing catch up but had to also make sure I was focusing on my recovery in the rest period. The workout just kept creeping away from me and unfortunately things didn't go to plan, I came fourteenth and I knew I had stuffed up big time.

"What were you thinking, Tia? You do realise what you've just done? Everything you've worked so hard for this entire weekend to create that buffer, you've just thrown it away and pissed it up against the wall in one workout."

I stared at Shane blankly. I was mad as anything and had no words. What he said was true.

"It's all down to the next workout, Tia. If you don't want to be second best again, then you've got to give it your all."

'Second best,' I thought, 'Like hell I'm going to be second best again, I'm leaving nothing out on the floor today'.

The end of the weekend was drawing near so there could only be one more event left. The CrossFit crew asked all of the athletes back out onto the competition floor for the announcement of the last workout. Then Dave announced the Fibonacci Final which consisted of: three parallette handstand push-ups; five kettlebell deadlifts, 124 pounds; five parallette handstand push-ups; eight kettlebell deadlifts, 124 pounds; eight parallette handstand push-ups; thirteen kettlebell deadlifts, 124 pounds. Then, lunge 89 feet with two 35 pound kettlebells overhead. It was make or break.

There was a lot of hype in the room once the workout was announced and I couldn't have been happier. You could see it all over my face; for a second I thought to myself, 'I have won.' I was so happy with the combination of movements - I love deadlifts, lunges and handstand push-ups. I was so geed up! 'I'm going to dominate this, there is no way Kara can beat me. This is my race, this is my Games.' I kept the voice in my head positive and remembered what Josh had said to me, 'Lesser people have won the Games, Tia, so why can't you?'

We were warming up for the movements just before the last workout and Shane was giving me his usual pep talk.

"Tia, it's not over until it's over. This is your event but don't get ahead of yourself. Make sure you stay focused, composed and play your own game. You have to beat Kara if you want to win the CrossFit Games."

"I have got this."

That's all I said and all I needed to say. I believed it was mine.

This buzzer started and after a couple of reps, my judge gave me a 'no rep' for my handstand push-ups, not just one 'no rep' but a few. He continued to make a few poor judgment calls throughout each of my sets, but I knew I couldn't let that cloud my focus. Those things happen in the heat of the moment, it's part of competition. But even with the 'no rep' calls I was still tracking ahead. I was six points ahead of Kara on the leaderboard so all I needed to do was keep the lead. I powered ahead in my lunges, each step closer to the finish line and the crowd got louder and louder. I got to the last couple of metres and panicked that Kara was right on my tail. I overstepped, which made me lose my overhead position and my left-hand kettlebell came down which meant I had to go back a metre. In that split-second Kara steamed through from behind and we crossed the finish line within milliseconds of each other. 'She got me,' I thought to myself. The crowd was cheering and the 2017 CrossFit Games was over.

***

Complete devastation. That's all I felt when I crossed that line. I looked over at Kara and she was trying to recover after such an epic fight. The screens flashed up and Kara beat me 3:47:80 to 3:47:99. I was furious with myself. I thought back to Shane saying, 'If you really want to win, then all you have to do is beat Kara', so all I thought to myself in that moment was, 'Well, I obviously don't want to win, I don't deserve to even be out here because I just gave it away AGAIN'. I didn't even want to face Shane, I was simply ashamed of my efforts, I felt like I hadn't learnt from the devastation last year and that I let it happen again so easily.

"I'm just not cut out to win."

I spoke to myself under my breath, I had never felt pain like it. I was so angry but I had to remind myself that the other girls were still crossing the line and I wanted to go and congratulate Kara on her amazing efforts. Despite my own frustration at myself, I was pleased for a fellow Australian to win. I was so happy for her.

The crowd was cheering so loudly, the atmosphere was electric. Once everyone was across the line from the final heat, the female competition was complete and the Games for us were over. There were tears of joy and relief from me and the other athletes. Relief that we had all made it through another year of the Games. However, I kept thinking, 'Tia, you idiot, you went to the Games to win.'

We all hugged and congratulated each other on an epic competition. Then Dave walked out onto the floor.

"Ladies and gentlemen, your 2017 Fittest on Earth is from Australia."

Dave asked for Kara and me to walk out on the floor together. I didn't want to go out as I didn't want to get in the way of Kara celebrating her win, it was her time. I hugged Kara one more time and congratulated her on her amazing efforts. We walked out together and I was very reluctant. Dave continued talking over the microphone.

"The 2017 Reebok CrossFit Games Champion is ..."

The pause was drawn out and the silence was deafening.

"... TIA-CLAIR TOOMEY!"

For a moment I thought Dave had made a mistake but then realised he was actually walking over to congratulate me and give me a hug. Then I thought, 'Maybe they gave it to me out of pity? How did I win? Kara beat me?'

But no one was correcting it. I collapsed and burst out crying, the emotion came pouring out of me. I WON! Kara gave me the biggest hug and congratulated me. I felt like she was genuinely happy for me too.

Once I hugged Kara, I made my way back to the crowd where Shane was standing. All I wanted to do was see Shane and embrace him in my arms. I tried to hold back my tears but they were uncontrollable, especially when I saw his face. I ran straight into his arms and squeezed him so tight.

"You did it, babe, you won!"

"We did it, we won."

"Now we can get married!"

"I can't believe we actually won, after all that hard work, you were right, Shane, it paid off and was so worth it."

"I'm so proud of you, babe, good job."

There were a lot of special moments throughout the Games but embracing Shane and sharing the win with him was without a doubt one of the best.

I ran back and hugged the rest of the girls all over again, crying and embracing the happy emotions. I truly felt like everyone was genuinely happy for me and that the whole stadium was in tears of joy alongside me. The girls hugged me and whispered their well wishes in my ear, 'Well done Tia, you really are the most deserving one for the top spot,' 'You are a great ambassador for this sport,' 'You are an incredible athlete and so deserving, congratulations.'

I was so honoured to hear everyone's kind words, especially from my very own competition. I just couldn't believe I actually did it. I fought so hard for the top spot and to come out on top was just the most incredible thing in the world.

I eventually found out that my heat was slow, which changed how all of the points were allocated. This meant I still finished at the top of the leaderboard but only by two points. I was a little disappointed for letting things run so tightly but a win is still a win and I couldn't have been happier.

That final event with Kara made me so proud to be Australian. We took everything we had to the 2017 Reebok CrossFit Games and we did it for ourselves and our country and became the people to beat. I am so excited for the 2018 Games. I want to go into the 2018 season being smarter and more dominating than ever before. Each year, my confidence and belief in myself grows. I won't be as conservative or cautious at the next Games, that confidence just comes with experience. The more experience and exposure I get, the more I learn about myself and understand how to deal with unexpected circumstances. At the 2017 Games, I pushed so hard in some of the events, to a point that I didn't even know I was capable of. Now I can't wait to see how much more my mind and body can give.

Marrying Shane in September, following my Games win, was the icing on the cake for me. All I could think was '2017 is my year!' When I married Shane, I felt so blessed to officially be a part of his beautiful family. Shane's Dad, Steve, is a caring and committed man who has always supported Shane and me. He welcomed me into the family like his very own daughter well before our wedding. When Shane and I first started dating, I remember Steve would constantly remind Shane not to distract me from school and was always there to help me. It was Steve who helped me get my driver's licence!

Shane's Mum, Myrna, is one of my biggest fans and is one of the most loving people on this planet. She is always checking in on me to see how I'm going and I always joke around and say that she loves me more than Shane. Coming from a family of girls, I always wanted brothers as well and I finally got my wish of having two of the best brothers anyone could ever ask for in Shane's brothers, Pat and Mat. I really am blessed to have my incredible family unit, I would be nothing without them.

***

Now it is back to the drawing board for me and I am focused on resetting my new goals for the future. I may have been the Fittest Woman on Earth in 2017 but come 2018, it's a new year and a new game; the leaderboard goes back to zero. I have had to work really hard to get to the top but in my eyes, real champions are made now. The real work begins in defending my title and staying on top.

I am currently training for the 2018 CrossFit Games season and the Commonwealth Games, which is like a mini Olympics for all the countries in the Commonwealth. My aim is to represent Australia in the 58kg category in weightlifting next April on the Gold Coast in Australia. Then it will be all eyes on the prize again for the 2018 CrossFit Games.

I hope you have enjoyed reading my journey so far, it has been a pleasure sharing it with you. I hope it has given you the motivation and encouragement to go out there and give your goals a go because now you know that I was just a normal person who was determined to achieve my dreams.

Anything is possible if you really want it.

MY FAVOURITE GREEN SM(O)THIE RECIPE

I can't start the day without my go-to Green Smoothie. It nourishes my body and boosts my immune system with lots of natural micro-nutrients.

- 250ml pure coconut water
- 2 handfuls of spinach leaves
- 1 carrot
- Half a cucumber
- Handful of blueberries
- 2 handfuls of kale leaves
- 2 handfuls of celery
- Thumb size of ginger
- Squeeze of lemon

Blend and enjoy!

HOW TO RECOVER LIKE A PRO

Training hard is a challenge in itself, but recovery is when the magic happens - when you recover properly, you're giving your body the opportunity to heal itself, rebuild damaged tissues and come back better for your next session.

SLEEP

Sleep is the most important variable for recovery. If you don't sleep long enough, with the right quality, you're not going to recover between workouts, your body will be sore and your mind sluggish. Simply put, unsatisfactory sleep will mean missing out on getting stronger, fitter and healthier. Sleep is the time your body dedicates to recovery, using stored resources to regenerate tissue, restore hormonal balance and recuperate mentally.

Over the past few months I've learned the value of good sleep and used it to drive my recovery. The minimum should be eight hours of sleep of the right quality. Maximising sleep quality requires sleeping in the darkest possible environment whilst being well-fed and hydrated. If you struggle to get to sleep, reduce 'screen-time' in the evening and if this doesn't work, consider a core circuit or mobility session followed by a glass of water – you'll soon be tired enough!

NUTRITION

Proper nutrition should be a cornerstone of every athlete's recovery. If your diet sucks it will be impossible to reach your goals - the structure of your diet is the basis for how you recover, progress and perform. Firstly, ensure you're eating enough – building muscle requires you to eat more calories than you use. If you're trying to get leaner, you'll want to do the opposite. The internet has loads of 'TDEE' calculators which will estimate your baseline calorie use. These aren't perfect, but they're a place to start. Once you've set your calorie balance, make sure you're getting the right balance of foods in a proper balance of dietary protein, carbohydrates and fats. This will improve your recovery further.

The needs of each individual are always slightly different, but a diet high in protein will make recovery much faster and easier, as well as aiding in both muscle growth and fat loss. However, this alone is not sufficient for optimal recovery; food quality plays a large role in health and performance. It's possible to achieve your calorie balance and macro-nutrients by eating junk food, but it is awful for recovery and health.

Junk foods are heavily processed and often low in micro-nutrients. Micro-nutrients (such as vitamins and minerals) are key for proper health and athletic performance through processes like energy transfer and protein synthesis, both of which are fundamental to strength and fitness. I keep it simple and give my body the best chance by sticking to whole foods wherever possible; cuts of meat, high-quality fish and lots of fruit and veg, which should be the cornerstone of any athletic diet!

Timing meals correctly will also improve your recovery. My rule of thumb is that food should be faster-absorbing closer to training. Breakfast and evening meals should consist of proteins and fats as well as some slow-digesting carbs. Meals that are a few hours away before and after training should be an even mixture of carbs, fats and protein and immediately before and after training, I like to focus on a combination of simple carbs and protein – this is usually in the form of a protein shake with fast-acting carbs to refuel after a tough session.

Training hard five to six days a week makes it difficult to hold onto body weight, but a proper approach to nutrition allows me to stay on top of my body. Building muscle whilst staying lean requires hard work and discipline in and out of the gym. Attention to detail in your diet will show in your performance.

HYDRATION

Staying hydrated is essential to health and performance. Proper water intake will make noticeable changes in general health, energy, muscular recovery and joint health. A bad session could be the result of failing to get enough water in while you rested - an easy fix. There are some obvious considerations; if you're training with high psychological intensity (it feels difficult), high volume or a lot of aerobic work then you're going to need a lot more water. However, your water intake outside of training is just as important - most people forget this because they're either busy or don't feel thirsty.

It's important to remember that not feeling thirsty is not the same as being well-hydrated. I always keep a bottle of water handy - you'd be amazed at how much more water you'll drink just by having it nearby, especially in the winter months.

MOBILITY

Mobility has received a lot of attention lately, for good reason - functioning as a human requires the flexibility to move well without pain. Training, especially hard or repetitive training, can cause all kinds of problems: joint impingement, connective tissue inflammation (tendonitis and others) and muscular tears, all of which can be reduced through mobility work.

Stretching and mobility work also reduces soreness and improves recovery after a tough training session. Mobility work has loads of components; stretching (both static and dynamic), foam rolling, flossing and massage are just some of the more popular methods. Dynamic stretching before a session helps to warm the joints, reduce impact injuries and improve exercise technique. Static stretching after or between sessions will help reduce DOMS and joint pain. Foam rolling will help remove waste products after exercise and is especially useful for endurance athletes. Massage is more expensive and sought-after for a reason - an experienced and knowledgeable sports massage therapist can reduce soreness, tightness and fix all the tension you accumulate over a long training career.

ACTIVE RECOVERY

Training for recovery is worth considering if you have the time and want to take your training seriously. Active recovery sessions are light, low-volume exercise aimed at accelerating the body's recovery responses. It might sound counterintuitive but your body doesn't want to be sat on the sofa - we're built to move every day and casual exercise will keep the blood flowing and de-stress the mind. Active recovery exercise can also be a great way to mix up your training and break the tediousness of training in the same environment. I like to drop the weights and get outdoors by walking, hiking or swimming. This won't be possible for everyone, but a quick pool session or walking through the park is an enjoyable way to commit some extra time to deliberate recovery.

SUMMARY

Recovery isn't going to make you a world-class athlete overnight or fix a bad approach to training. However, it is a tool at your disposal to become the best athlete you can and keep coming back at your best. If you spend dozens of hours in the gym every week then a few hours out of the gym, focusing on how you treat your body, is a relatively small task. Adding even a few of these methods should make a real difference in the way you feel and perform. Training hard is a challenge itself, but recovery is when the magic happens. When you recover properly, you're helping yourself become better than what you were yesterday.

EATING & WEIGHT LOSS FOR OPTIMAL HEALTH

A MACROS APPROACH TO EATING

I have tried multiple nutrition plans and diets but all have left me consuming either too much food or not enough food. Now I follow a macros approach to eating where I track my carbohydrates, fats and proteins. This ensures I eat the right portion sizes and types of food for my body to perform at its best.

My current macros are:
Proteins: 140g
Carbohydrates: 235g
Fats: 55g

These macros help me maintain a consistent body weight of 60kg. This is heavy enough for my CrossFit training and light enough so that when I need to cut weight for weightlifting, I can easily reduce to 58kg with only a few small changes.

I don't eat a specific number of macros for breakfast, lunch and dinner. I choose to space my required macros throughout the day, ensuring my intake complements my training schedule. My macros coach is a lady named Adee from Working Against Gravity. When Dee writes my meal plan, she always provides me with a refeed day, where I eat extra carbohydrates to get my body ready for the following week of dieting. This allows me to restore glycogen stores and get over any adaptations that may occur in my body from dieting. It also gives me a day where I can make certain foods fit into my macros that I wouldn't usually have. Psychologically, this helps keep me on track as I am able to indulge a little bit.

Why I like following a macro approach to eating:
· I can consume a larger variety of foods which is beneficial when I'm travelling.
· I can still go out with friends and enjoy a meal.
· I am more aware of the importance of micro-nutrition in food.
· I am able to easily manage my body weight for weightlifting competitions.

DROPPING WEIGHT FOR
WEIGHTLIFTING

I thought I'd share a little example of what my macros coach gets me to do when I'm cutting weight for my weightlifting competitions.

The amount of water I consume five days before competition is critical. The amount of water can vary depending on the athlete but this is a sample of what I follow:

- Five days out - consume 2 gallons
- Four days out - consume 1 gallon
- Three days out - consume 1 gallon
- Two days out - consume .5 gallons
- One day out - consume .25 gallons
- Weigh-in day - no water until after weigh-in

When cutting weight, my macros would look very similar to this:

Two weeks out with a body weight of 60kg:
- Protein: 140g
- Carbohydrates: 230g
- Fats: 50g

One week out with a body weight of 59.5kg:
- Protein: 140g
- Carbohydrates: 220g
- Fats: 55g

Three days out with a body weight of 59kg:
- Protein: 140g
- Carbohydrates: 180g
- Fats: 60g

Two days out with a body weight of 58.5kg:
- Protein: 140g
- Carbohydrates: 175g
- Fats: 60g

One day out with a body weight of 58kg:
- Protein: 140g
- Carbohydrates: 175g
- Fats: 60g

Game day with a body weight of 57.5kg:
- On game day, I don't stick to macros. I weigh myself with food in my hand to ensure I know exactly how much weight I will put on as a result of eating that food. Generally, I will eat a few slices of bread with jam or honey because it doesn't weigh much and satisfies my hunger while I wait for weigh-in.

When I embark on losing weight for a competition, I make sure I time the process correctly. I allow enough time to cut down on portion sizes so that the process is gentle on my body. It is not good for me to drop weight too fast or too slow because it affects my energy and recovery levels.

I always weigh in two hours before my session starts so as soon as I have checked in, registered my starting weight and weighed in, I try and rehydrate my body as quickly as possible.

The food I generally have after weigh-in includes:
- 2 bottles of Powerade
- 1 bottle of water
- 1 banana
- Ham and salad sandwich with a white bread bun
- I will also have a pack of Allen's Snakes (candy) for Shane, Miles and myself to snack on throughout competition

Information provided by Adee from Working Against Gravity

This is the weight loss process I follow when I'm working with Tia.

Cutting weight for a weightlifting meet is a little bit trickier because the number on the scale becomes very important. When Tia trains for CrossFit, her weight is important but it does not need to be as precise. In the weeks leading up to a weightlifting meet, I monitor nutrition much more closely in an attempt to maximise calorie consumption while also reducing body weight so that Tia can compete in her desired weight class. My goal is to limit any extreme measures like spitting, sweating, sauna or complete calorie restriction so that training does not suffer, recovery can still occur, and psychologically there is not too much stress.

For every gram of carbohydrates, everyone's body needs to hold onto three grams of water. This means that carbohydrates can cause temporary weight gain. The weeks before a meet I am trying to avoid any extra water retention, so cutting down carbohydrates is always my first step if weight is not coming down quickly enough. I will check in daily with Tia to make sure

body weight is moving in the right direction. It is important to track body weight before going to sleep, as well as body weight in the morning so I can get a good idea of how much weight Tia loses overnight (this is called "float" weight). This way we can know exactly how much Tia needs to weigh going to sleep the night before weigh-in, potentially even allowing her to eat the following morning.

If necessary, one last minute technique I will use with Tia is to manipulate water. This is NOT suggested for the average lifter. If you aren't competing in weightlifting, then cutting weight to this extreme should not be a priority.

Cutting weight with water is a simple and effective way to drop the number on the scale without needing to cut as many calories. How does this work? Well, when you drink excessive amounts of water your body will go into a "flushing mode". This happens because our bodies have increased the mechanisms to promote water loss. More water in, equals more water out. Drinking more water will also cause the body to lower both

aldosterone and ADH (Antidiuretic Hormone), the two primary hormones involved in urine production and water secretion from the body. These lower levels of Aldosterone will promote increased water loss.

When you increase water intake, the increase in urine output does not happen instantly. Aldosterone and ADH are slow to respond. As you continue to keep your water intake high, you will start to see those hormones respond, urine output will increase and body weight will drop. This lag in response also occurs when we decrease water intake. This means water loss remains high even with very little water intake. Most people can see this trend continue for 72+ hours before ADH and Aldosterone catch on and levels start to increase, causing water retention. Athletes can lose from 5-15lbs this way.

REMEMBER — this is an extreme way to cut weight and may leave you feeling like you have lower energy levels.

STAYING MOTIVATED

I USE A NUMBER OF TOOLS TO KEEP ME MOTIVATED THROUGHOUT THE YEAR, ESPECIALLY IN THE OFF SEASON. IT IS IMPORTANT TO KEEP MYSELF IN A POSITIVE FRAME OF MIND, ESPECIALLY BECAUSE THE CROSSFIT GAMES IS JUST AS MUCH A MENTAL GAME AS IT IS A PHYSICAL ONE.

1. Positive self-talk and simple motivational quotes are tools I draw on to help me avoid negative thoughts and self-doubt. I enjoy writing down and printing off sayings that I come across which relate to and resemble my own personal drive and determination in some way. I like to learn some of them off by heart and say them to myself when I'm preparing to complete. They definitely help me get to the top of the podium.

2. The expression "GOOD" is one of my favourites and I thank Josh Bridges for sharing this one with me. Whenever something is hard or challenging or whenever I'm in pain, I tell myself it's a good thing, and it is because it means I'm pushing hard and getting better!

3. I often think back to when my Dad would tuck me into bed at night and I would ask him, "Do you think I did enough at training today?" Dad would reply, "If you can lay here knowing you gave it absolutely everything you had to give today, then you did enough but if there is something that you think you could have done better, then you know you need to work harder." It's so simple, but so true and I never leave anything on the floor.

4. I like the principle of 'Feeding the Good Wolf.' It speaks to the idea that we all have two wolfs inside of us – a good and a bad. The good wolf is positive and beneficial, while the bad wolf is negative and destructive. The wolf that wins is the wolf we feed so always try to feed the good one!

5. Something Shane often says to me when I'm struggling is, "The harder you work today, the easier it will be in competition." I know this to be true and it reaffirms to me that hard work will pay off and the blood, sweat and tears ARE worth it.

6. 'Keeping the balance' is paramount to me achieving my goals. Taking my dogs to the beach, going to the movies with Shane, going out to dinner with friends, watching trashy shows on Netflix are all things I love to do to recharge my mind and body. This enables me to have a life outside of training and resets my mind so I can be 100% focused and energised.

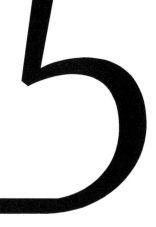

REASONS TO SQUAT

Squatting plays a major role in my CrossFit and weightlifting training. I know that if I've got great squat numbers, I'm going to have great performances. My own training routine includes squatting a minimum of three times per week, mixing up both front and back squats as needed. Here's a little list of the top five reasons squatting is so important to me:

BUILDING MUSCLE AND OVERALL STRENGTH

Squatting is a foundational movement! It is a completely natural movement which works the muscles of the back, quads, hamstrings, core, and calves. Practicing squats keeps those muscles, and the joints they articulate on, strong and mobile. I maintain a strict squatting routine to build that foundation of strength and muscle, which is what keeps me performing at my best. Building muscle mass is not really a priority for me in either weightlifting or CrossFit. This is because weighing less is actually one of my advantages. As long as I can maintain the level of strength I have built and my strength isn't compromised by my weight, I will stay consistently close to the weight I am at the moment. However, a certain amount of mass is necessary to increase

strength and there will always be some mass that gets packed on by default when doing volume training, I just make sure it isn't too much! Overall, strength is really what I am after and without the functional strength I get from squatting, I wouldn't be performing at the high level that I do.

FUNCTIONALITY AND UTILITY

Squatting is totally natural, we know that, so let's talk more about why I really need to squat to perform. It's one of the most functional parts of CrossFit; we see squatting in all the lifts; as well as wall ball, box jumps and many more movements.
The foundation of a good squat number and the mobility to perform front, back and overhead squats correctly goes a long way. When I started out, a 1RM squat of 80kg would only get me so far... having a sizeable squat helps make all the other movements less intensified and more manageable.

STRONG CORRELATION TO WEIGHTLIFTING

It's pretty obvious to say, but any lifter performs heaps of squats. The strength power in my back and legs to move weights around requires a lot of squatting. After all, a clean is truly dependent upon whether you can stand up with that bar or not. Lifters typically squat three to five times per week at varying intensities and volumes, often staying in the 2RM to 5RM range.

IMPROVEMENT IN SPRINTING

Back squats are always a favourite for sprint athletes

and it's no different for me. It requires us to explode, with as much power as possible and using the exact same chain of muscles, in the same sequence as sprinting, though unilaterally. I don't want to say that squatting itself makes me faster, because that would be inaccurate to some degree but squatting definitely makes you stronger. The definition of "power" is the change in speed over time. So, squatting allows me to generate the strength needed to improve my power. Again, a foundation of strength is the most important part of your body that will help you perform better in all aspects. Side note: A great exercise that I implement is jumping barbell squats. This has helped my power and my ability to be more explosive, particularly at the start of races.

IMPROVEMENT IN CORE STRENGTH

All of the movements are initiated in the core. Think of walking, running, lifting and all of the overhead movements I need to do in CrossFit. All the planks and sit-ups in the world couldn't strengthen my core like squats do.
The oblique and transverse abdominals are stabilised through squats as the load is placed at the top of the spine, forcing it to maintain an upright position. The mechanics of a front squat puts even more stress on the core as the weight is shifted anterior, creating a longer lever to force through. Front squats work my core in the most functional way possible, because it replicates exactly the strength I need for cleans, wall balls and thrusters, as well as a lot of the overhead work.

ACHIEVING
YOUR GOALS

Whether your goals are recreational or competitive, to look better on the beach or on the competition stage, you have to set yourself up for success by approaching it with the right mentality and making the most of your time. Here's how I make the most of my training and push myself to progress.

Firstly, you have to push yourself to train smarter. When I step into the gym, I'm there to train, not just to exercise. If you want to get better at something then your hard work has to be focused on improving. This sounds really simple and obvious but it means that you don't just turn up to the gym, do the work and go home; you have to focus on what details you need to work on. For example, if you know that your snatch is a weakness then you need to turn up to training with ideas about what you're going to do to improve on that day and be deliberate and intentional in your training. If you just do your working sets and go home then you may have put in the work but your technique isn't going to improve – this is the same in any of the components of CrossFit and weightlifting. A good coach is a huge help - sometimes it's hard to know what you should be working on, which makes it easy to work on nothing and just cruise through workouts. If you have a great coach or training partner who can spur you on with some technical feedback, you'll make much faster progress. I am very fortunate that I have a great coach in Shane who does everything with me and is constantly giving me feedback.

Secondly, it is important to know from the very start that you will encounter some obstacles to your progress. Setbacks will occur and you have to have the right mentality towards them or you'll only get yourself down. It's easy to get demotivated after an injury or when the general stress and pressure gets to you. If you're working long hours, have family commitments or a bout of poor health that is affecting your training, then you have to remember WHY you train in the first place and see it as a short-term problem. In the grand scheme of things, a few weeks or even months where you can't prioritise your training or have to train around other commitments won't ruin your performance forever. Even elite athletes get injured, putting them out for months at a time, but they still come back stronger than ever and compete on the world's biggest platforms. You have to have that same mentality if you want to progress; setbacks will happen but they have to only set you back rather than totally derail you. Taking a long-term view of your training is hard but it will help keep everything in perspective.

The long-term view of training also means that we have to approach training goals properly. Most people have a big goal that they have set for themselves. It might be to lose 10kg in the next six months or add 30kg to a back squat or taking minutes off a benchmark workout. However, these big goals can be blinding if you don't approach them properly. If your goal is to lose weight in the next six months, there's plenty of time to 'do it later!' To achieve a goal, you have to have a sense of urgency in your training and what you're eating; otherwise you'll find yourself stagnating and making excuses for not progressing. This is why you need to have intermediate goals. Intermediate goals are the smaller goals that you put between yourself and your long-term goal to keep the goal present and keep yourself motivated. If we look at it like we are closing the distance between where we are now and where we want to be, we can avoid feeling like our goals are impossibly large and are actually achievable.

Examples of this are varied: we might set our short-term weight loss goal as losing 1kg in the next two weeks, squatting a PR set of 5 or improving our technique in one of the components of our favourite benchmark workout. These are all steps in the right direction and will keep your training and eating focused, effective and rewarding. Achieving your goals won't just happen and you can't be passive about your training. Whether you want to lose weight, gain muscle or perform at your best, you have to make it happen. If you stick to a deliberate approach to training, accept that setbacks will come but they won't break you and structure your training so that small improvements are your focus. You'll soon find that you've made big progress.

CORE STRENGTH
GIVES YOU GAINS

When I refer to core strength, I'm not referring to the aesthetic look of making and maintaining a six pack. That would be of no significant value to me, since looking a certain way has no bearing on my training.

I need a core that is capable of handling huge loads from movements like squats, yoke carry, and high reps of toes to bar or GHD sit-ups and so on. When it comes to weightlifting, strong legs just won't cut it. I need a core that can withstand nearly twice my bodyweight an arm-length overhead. Every movement I do is initiated by the muscles of the core. Without a strong core, you can expect hip, back or shoulder pain, along with a strength plateau in many exercises. Think of a tree standing up against a cyclone; a horizontal force placed at the very top of the structure, catching the wind. Those with stronger, thicker trunks can withstand immense force and won't topple over. But the thinner, weaker trunks will simply give out. The trunk of our bodies functions in much the same way.

This concept is also referred to as "core to extremity" by many CrossFit coaches. We need that core to be as strong as possible as it bridges together the extremities. Overhead movements aren't the only ones that require strong core stability. Any movement in front or back racks like lunges, squats, dumbbell work or even strength work like bent over rows or good mornings all require a strong core. The core works in two ways. First, it stabilises our bodies in an upright position. This uses the three muscle layers of the abs - the transverse abdominals, which are deepest and run horizontally, the obliques, which run diagonally (superior-laterally to inferio-medially), and the rectus abdominus, which run vertically. All of them need to function in a perfect ratio to ensure I have the best core stability through all my lifts.

We also can't forget the importance of the quadratus lumborum and pelvic floor muscles. All of the core muscles support and stabilize the pelvis and spine, allowing a functional unit. A stable core will mean that the position of the spine is maintained and a vertical spine is a happy spine! Whether upright or hinged at the hip, a strong core will maintain the rigidity in my trunk and allow me to perform technical lifts correctly and safely.

A deficiency in any of the abdominal muscles or overall weakness could leave me being unstable overhead or unable to maintain correct posture through a pull or through a recovery during the clean. A weak core can lead to knee, hip, back and shoulder pain. Again, we talk about how the core links the extremities, and this is an example of why a person might be experiencing shoulder pain with weak abs. To prevent injury, maintaining a strong core is vital. I see a lot of people pinch their belly fat (or skin) and say, 'oh, I have literally NO abs!' Of course, this would be completely impossible if they are able to stand or sit up. What

they are probably referring to is not having definition, which comes down to nutrition, and whether someone is very defined doesn't seem to effect lifting or CrossFit performance!

In the same way, a flat stomach is not necessarily indicative of a strong core or a healthy body. Rather than deciding to work on your core because you want a bikini body, base it on science. Experiment with your lifts and see if you can figure out what is limiting your movements. If you break form easily and it is initiated in the core area, you have your answer! If you have perfect posture through squats and pressing but feel it in the lower or upper limbs, you might be just fine with your current core strength. A good coach or a fellow lifter might be able to help you out using a video so you can get visual feedback of your mechanics and how you move. A strong core can really make or break you as an athlete. If you find you do have a weak core, strengthening it will give you big gains in your lifts.

I have an eight-week core program that you can follow if you head to my website tiaclair.com. You can purchase it online and do exactly what I do to help your core strength!

I would like to thank everyone who has helped me throughout my CrossFit & Weightlifting career thus far. You all know who you are and I want you to know that your time and effort has not gone unnoticed and that I am forever grateful. All the sacrifices you have made in order to help me achieve my dreams is the reason I am where I am today. It is because of you that I keep going back to the gym and giving 110% effort every day. Thank you from the bottom of my heart, I love you all so much and I hope I can continue to make you proud. Here is to the future xo

Special thanks to WODproof for their ongoing support.

Tia-Clair Toomey

Tia-Clair